Nutrition Essentials
5th Edition

A Guidebook for the
Fitness Professional

Joe Cannon, MS

FauldHouse Publishing

Joe Cannon's Websites: Joe-Cannon.com **AND** Supplement-Geek.com

Printed in the United States of America
Published November 2014

Table of Contents

For Mom & Dad

May there be libraries in heaven...

Acknowledgments

I have always felt that we are truly blessed by the quality of the people whom we can count among our friends. I have been blessed by some friends whom I would like to formally thank now, who assisted me in various capacities during the creation of this book.

Many thanks also to Kelly Bixler and Dianna Mills, MS, who were instrumental in sharing both their unique insights and editing skills.

Thank you to Bill Leinhauser, Timothy DiFelice, and Adam Freedman for their continued encouragement, reassurance, and friendship over the years.

I would also like to thank everyone who is an owner of previous editions of *Nutrition Essentials*. Your faith in me as a writer and educator has been an inspiration and played a key role in my decision to refine this book to further meet the nutrition and personal training needs of fitness professionals.

What's This Book About?

With the first edition of Nutrition Essentials, I began my quest to bring to the fitness professional a resource where she or he could read concise and up-to-date information on a myriad of nutrition- and fitness-related topics and issues commonly encountered in the wellness field. This book builds upon the previous editions by providing additional information to help broaden the knowledge of readers.

Since writing this book, I've started blogging about health, fitness and wellness. So, in this 5th edition of the book, where appropriate, I'll mention related blogs posts I've written where people can go to get more information.

As with past editions, I had two main goals when writing this book. First, I wanted to create a text that would help fitness professionals cut through the sometimes murky and complicated waters that seem to permeate our field. Second, I wanted to present a text that explains complex topics in easy to understand language. It's likely that many of you have a large library of wellness-related books. Some of those books, however, explain things in complex and technical language. *Nutrition Essentials* was written to help bridge that gap and to foster greater understanding on the part of the reader. This can be particularly invaluable for those studying for a certification and who want answers fast.

Every chapter is independent of the others, so you can start anywhere you like. I have also included a glossary of terms at the end of the book to further assist with researching and understanding the major topics presented in the text. In addition, a detailed index is included to help people quickly jump to the area for which they are looking.

It is my hope that you will find value in *Nutrition Essentials*. Comments are always welcome and you can reach me through my websites.

Joe Cannon

www.Joe-Cannon.com

Chapter 1

The Macronutrients

The term *macro* means "big." Macronutrients are molecules from which we can obtain energy and which are also nutritious, providing vitamins, minerals, fiber, and other important elements needed to stay healthy. Macronutrients are also consumed in greater quantities than other nutrients. There are three macronutrients: *carbohydrates*, *fats*, and *proteins*. Below is a brief review of the macronutrients, along with other relevant issues with which fitness professionals should be familiar.

Carbohydrate

The term *carbohydrate* is another name for sugar. Carbohydrates (carbs) were given this name because they all contain the elements carbon, hydrogen, and oxygen.[36] Examples of carbohydrates include bread, rice, potatoes, glucose (blood sugar), lactose (milk sugar), broccoli, and other vegetables. Most carbohydrates in the human diet are derived from plants.[36] Carbohydrates can be subdivided into the following types of molecules: monosaccharides, disaccharides, oligosaccharides, and polysaccharides. Each name is related to the number of sugars that make up the molecule in question. For example, monosaccharides are single sugar molecules, while disaccharides are composed of two sugar molecules linked together. Polysaccharides are composed of many sugar molecules.

Polysaccharides

Polysaccharides are composed of several thousand sugar molecules chemically bonded together. Examples of polysaccharides include starch, glycogen, and fiber, to name a few.

- **Starch.** Starch is the carbohydrate storage molecule of plants. Starch is found in foods such as spaghetti, rice, cereal, and bread.

- **Glycogen.** Glycogen forms the stored sugar reserves in animals and humans. It is found in both the muscle, where it serves as a direct energy source to the muscles during activity, and the liver, where it allows for an even regulation of blood sugar levels between meals. Glycogen is produced from the bonding together of many glucose molecules during the process called *glucogenesis* and is broken down through the process called *glycogenolysis*.[36] Thus, glucose and glycogen are essentially different forms of the same molecule. As will be discussed later, broken-down glycogen, along with fats, serves as a major nutrient used for fuel during aerobic exercise. Glycogen is often called the *limiting factor* because when one runs out of glycogen, exercise stops. Runners sometimes call this phenomenon *hitting the wall*. The average person has between 1,500 and 2,000 calories of glycogen stored in his or her body—enough energy to power a 20-mile run at high speed.[36]

Fiber

Fiber is a general term used to describe indigestible plant structures.[26] Found only in plants, fiber gives bulk to food and helps people feel full.[37] In terms of weight control, fiber may help prevent weight gain and obesity by reducing the number of calories consumed. While the typical American obtains roughly 12–15 grams of fiber daily, the recommended dietary allowance (RDA) for fiber is 25–35 grams per day.[26]

Fiber can be divided into both *water-soluble* fiber and *water-insoluble* fiber. Studies show that water-soluble fiber such as pectin and oats can modestly reduce blood cholesterol levels.[26] Water-insoluble fiber does not have cholesterol-lowering effects but may offer other healthy benefits.[36]

In addition to reducing obesity and cholesterol levels, fiber also contains other nutrients beneficial to health. For example, fiber contains magnesium, which may play a role in alleviating some symptoms of diabetes.[26] Examples of high-fiber foods include whole-wheat pasta, brown rice, oatmeal, and vegetables. For this reason, nutrition professionals frequently counsel people to increase their intake of these foods.

Fiber and Health

Dietary fiber has recently received much attention because of research showing that increasing fiber intake reduces one's risk of various diseases. Epidemiological studies of large numbers of people have shown that people who consume the most fiber tend to be less likely to develop diabetes, obesity, heart disease, high blood pressure, and intestinal disorders than those who consume less.[46, 47] Theories abound as to how fiber-rich diets protect us from these disorders. While one such theory suggests that added fiber may decrease the amount of time that harmful materials remain in the body, another proposes that fiber may dilute and/or bind toxins, reducing the chance that they can cause problems in the body. A third theory holds that fiber may result in a scraping or scrubbing action that might dislodge harmful substances from the gastrointestinal tract to prevent them from doing harm.[36] Fiber may even perform all of these functions as well as others which have yet to be determined.

Throughout the world, carbohydrates comprise a large percentage of daily caloric intakes. In the typical American diet, for example, carbohydrates make up between 40 and 50% of daily calories. For individuals who exercise, this percentage may need to be increased to about 60%.[36]

Contrary to popular belief, all carbohydrates are not created equal. Carbohydrates from processed foods such as cookies, cakes, and other snack foods, known as *simple carbs*, are not equivalent to the *complex carbohydrates* found in fruits, vegetables, and whole grains. Not only do complex carbohydrates contain fewer calories than processed foods, but they are also rich in water, vitamins, minerals, fiber, and phytonutrients. Thus, when possible, people should strive to emphasize fruits, vegetables, and whole grains while avoiding candy, soda, cookies, or cakes.

Lactose Intolerance

Some people do not have the ability to digest milk sugar (lactose). Specifically, these individuals lack an enzyme called *lactase*, which breaks down lactose. For lactose intolerant individuals, consumption of milk or other lactose-containing dairy products may result in cramping and other gastrointestinal symptoms. Over-the-counter products and lactose-free foods are available to help these individuals eat a healthy, well rounded diet.

Carbohydrates and Exercise

As mentioned previously, carbohydrates are essential active individuals because they are a *rate-limiting fuel*. In other words, once carbohydrate stores are depleted, exercise performance decreases dramatically. Simply stated, nobody wins a marathon eating a low-carbohydrate diet.

Carbohydrates are used in greater amounts as exercise intensity increases.[36] Because high intensity activities with a short duration require quick energy, they require more carbohydrates for fuel than more moderate forms of exercise. For example, running a 5-minute mile uses a greater percentage of carbohydrates than running a 15-minute mile.

Carbohydrates and Ketones

Carbohydrates are essential for burning fat because byproducts from carbohydrate metabolism are needed to properly break down body fat.[36] The absence of carbs ramps up the protein breakdown and increases the body's production of *ketones*. While ketones are normally made in small amounts, production is increased during low-carb diets so that they may be used for fuel when carbohydrates are not available. However, because they are acidic in nature, prolonged periods of elevated ketones may cause *ketosis*, a condition that can be fatal, especially for those with pre-existing medical issues.

Fat

Fat reserves serve as the most abundant source of energy in the body.[36] In fact, the average adult male stores between 50,000 and 100,000 calories of energy as fat.[36] Also called *lipids*, fats consist of long chains of carbon atoms surrounded by hydrogen atoms.

Contrary to popular belief, fats serve a variety of important functions in the body and are an important component of a healthy diet. Not only do fats make up key cellular components of every cell membrane in the body, but they also insulate the body to protect it from cold temperatures, provide shock absorption for crucial organs to prevent damage, and form components of numerous molecules essential for the body to function properly. Fat is also an excellent source of energy, with each gram of fat containing 9 calories. While this may not seem significant, consider that the average person's body fat supplies enough energy for a non-stop run lasting about 120 hours![36] Still, because fats may contribute to the development of diseases and syndromes ranging from heart disease and some forms of cancer to diabetes, obesity, and many more, consumption of this nutrient should be moderate. Experts recommend that fat should comprise less than 30% of an individual's daily caloric intake.

Aside from being the long-term energy-storage molecule of the body, fat also acts as an important source of calories during long-duration activities such as running a marathon. While fat mobilization begins almost as soon as exercise begins, it does not represent a major contributor to one's energy needs at the start of exercise. As exercise continues, however, the body uses an increased percentage of fat. In other words, fat serves as a significant fuel source during any low intensity, long-duration activity.

Calories of the Macronutrients	
Macronutrient	Calorie per gram
• Carbohydrate	4
• Protein	4
• Fat	9

The table above provides a quick overview of the calories contained in each of the macronutrients. As can be seen, both carbohydrate and protein each contain 4 calories per gram. Fat, on the other hand, contains 9 calories per gram. Looking at this from another point of view, if all three macronutrients weighed equally, fat would have two and a half times as many calories as either carbohydrate or protein. This fact has profound implications for weight loss. By limiting fat in the diet, one may substantially limit the number of calories consumed. Ultimately, consuming fewer calories than one burns leads to weight loss. This is why people frequently report weight loss when following low-fat diets.

Triglycerides

Triglyceride is yet another name for fat. Triglycerides are not only the most abundant fat in the body, but also represent the major storage form of fat.[36] Triglycerides are stored within specialized cells called *adipose cells* or fat cells.

Saturated vs. Unsaturated Fats

As stated previously, fats consist of long chains of carbon atoms surrounded by hydrogen atoms. The number of hydrogen atoms which surround the carbon chain of a particular fat determines whether it is saturated or unsaturated.

In *saturated fats*, every available attachment point on the carbon chain is occupied by a hydrogen atom. Thus, they are literally *saturated* with hydrogen atoms, which alters the fat's chemical properties. Research suggests that diets high in saturated fats may increase one's risk of developing heart disease. Animal products such as beef, dairy products, and some foods derived from plants, such as coconut and palm oils, tend to be high in saturated fat.[36] Cookies, cakes, pies, and similar commercially-produced items are also a source of saturated fats. On food labels, saturated fats may be identified by two alternate names—*hydrogenated* or *partially hydrogenated* oils. Generally, saturated fats are usually easily recognized because they are solid at room temperature. Experts recommend that people eat no more than 10 percent of daily calories in the form of saturated fat.[36]

Unsaturated fats are said to be more "heart-healthy" than saturated fats. Generally, unsaturated fats are obtained from plant–based foods and are typically liquid at room temperature. Despite the fact that unsaturated fats have more health benefits than saturated fats, it is important to remember that both have 9 calories per gram and can lead to weight gain if consumed in excess. Unsaturated fats can be further sub-divided according to their degree of saturation with hydrogen. For example, an unsaturated fat that has one space unoccupied by a hydrogen atom is called *monounsaturated*, while an unsaturated fat with many spaces unoccupied by hydrogen atoms is termed *polyunsaturated*.

Food Sources of Fats	
Type of Fat	**Sources**
• Saturated Fat	butter, whole milk, coconut oil, palm oil
• Polyunsaturated Fat	evening primrose oil, flaxseed, tuna, safflower oil
• Monounsaturated Fat	peanuts, olive oil, canola oil

What Are Trans Fatty Acids?

Trans fatty acids have a different molecular arrangement than do saturated or unsaturated fats. Trans fatty acids are formed during *hydrogenation*, the process of making saturated fats, and tend to be found in processed foods such as cakes, cookies, and fried foods. Some studies have shown that trans fats can reduce good cholesterol (HDL), and raise bad cholesterol (LDL), which may increase one's risk for heart disease.[51] Other research notes that women whose bodies contain high levels of trans fatty acids are about 40% more likely to develop breast cancer than women with lower levels of trans fatty acids.[36] Preliminary research stemming mostly from laboratory animals hints that diets high in trans fats may reduce testosterone levels.[68] The implications of this for humans requires further study, and the role that trans fatty acids play in the development of various diseases is still being investigated. Fortunately, identifying foods that contain these fats is relatively easy. Foods whose labels use the terms *hydrogenated* or *partially hydrogenated* tend to contain trans fats. Thus, limiting consumption of hydrogenated and partially hydrogenated fats also limits ingestion of trans fats. Because of the link between trans fats and diseases such as cancer, heart disease, and more, food labels in the U.S. are required to explicitly list trans fats as well.

Cholesterol

Cholesterol is a lipid found only in animal tissues.[36] In humans, cholesterol can be ingested through cholesterol-containing foods or produced naturally in the liver. Though too much cholesterol can be harmful to one's health, the lipid serves several very important functions. For example, cholesterol is a component of every cell membrane in the human body, helping cells to maintain integrity. Cholesterol is also integral for the production of testosterone, estrogen, and vitamin D.

In spite of its crucial role in health, too much cholesterol can contribute to many health problems. Because heart disease risk tends to increase as blood cholesterol concentrations increase, experts recommend maintaining a relatively low total cholesterol level, preferably less than 200 milligrams per deciliter (mg/dL). Sometimes those with high cholesterol levels try to control it by eating fewer cholesterol-containing foods. However, because the body also makes cholesterol, this strategy may or may not work, as the body may compensate for the reduction in dietary cholesterol by making more in the liver. Given the health benefits of reducing levels of cholesterol in the blood, those who have elevated levels of the lipid are advised to work with their physician or dietitian to make the necessary dietary changes. Just a one percent reduction in cholesterol levels reduces heart disease risk by 2%, so working to develop healthy eating habits is well worth the effort.[36]

Besides cholesterol itself, two types of cholesterol—HDL and LDL—are also important for overall heart health. HDL and LDL are known as *good* and *bad* cholesterol, respectively. Let's review each briefly here and describe what they do.

- **HDL.** HDL stands for *high-density lipoprotein.* HDL transports excess cholesterol back to the liver, where it is recycled. HDL is commonly referred to as *good* cholesterol because it removes excess cholesterol from the bloodstream, reducing its chances of being incorporated into artery-clogging plaque. Foods don't contain HDL—the body makes it naturally. It is recommended that HDL levels be greater than or equal to 40 mg/dL for men and 50 mg/dL for women. An HDL level of 60 or better is considered a *negative risk factor* for heart disease, as HDL clears excess cholesterol from the blood to reduce its chances of building up.[2] Studies show that exercise can raise HDL levels in many individuals.

- **LDL.** LDL stands for *low-density lipoprotein* and is the so-called *bad* cholesterol. LDL transports cholesterol from the liver, where it is made, to the cells of the body, which use cholesterol in a variety of ways, such as producing testosterone and vitamin D. Because high blood cholesterol levels are associated with heart disease, elevated levels of LDL may theoretically transport more cholesterol than the body needs, resulting in the build-up of cholesterol in blood vessels and the formation of artery-clogging plaque. On blood tests, LDL should be less than 100 mg/dL although it could be lower for those with heart disease. Studies show that exercise may lower LDL in some individuals.

Accepted Blood Lipid Levels	
Lipid	**Accepted Level (mg/dl)**
Cholesterol	Less than 200
HDL	Greater than 40
LDL	Less than 100
Triglycerides	Less than 150

What about Cholesterol Ratios?

When cholesterol is checked by a doctor, one of the calculations usually performed is the *total cholesterol to HDL ratio.* This is sometimes abbreviated as *CHOL/HDL risk ratio.* This number is calculated by dividing the total cholesterol by the HDL. For example, if your total cholesterol is 150 mg/dL and your HDL level is 60 mg/dL, the ratio will be 150 ÷ 60, or 2.5. Keeping the CHOL/HDL risk ratio below 5 is one way to reduce the risk of developing heart disease. For every full–number decrease in this ratio (for example, going from 5 to 4), the risk of heart disease drops by 50%.[38]

Another ratio you may see is the *LDL to HDL ratio,* which tells how much LDL is present in relation to how much HDL is in the blood. It is calculated by dividing the LDL number by the HDL number. Low risk is between 0.5 to 3.0, while high risk is 6.0 or more.

A third ratio is called the triglyceride to HDL ratio. With this, you divide HDL into triglyceride level. For example, if your triglycerides are 100 and HDL is 50, your ratio is

100 ÷ 50, or 2. A ratio of 2 or less is considered *good,* while a ratio of 4 or above may increase heart disease risk.

Protein

Aside from being one of the main constituents of muscle tissue, protein forms a wide variety of molecules in the body. Some have estimated that proteins comprise over 50,000 different compounds in the human body.[36] Individual properties of each of these protein-containing structures are determined by the sequence of amino acids—the building blocks of proteins. Humans require 20 different amino acids to make all of the different protein structures found in the body. By changing the order or arrangement of amino acids, it is possible to make different proteins that serve different functions and have different properties. This is similar to the way that words are formed. Though there are only 26 letters in the English alphabet, those letters can form hundreds of thousands of words. Different arrangements of letters make various words, just as different arrangements of amino acids make various proteins. Good sources of protein include chicken, turkey, whey, soy, beef, and tuna, to name a few. The amino acids that make up proteins can be further broken down into essential amino acids and non-essential amino acids, which are discussed below.

Essential & Non-Essential Amino Acids

Essential amino acids are those that must be obtained from eating food or taking supplements. The *non-essential amino acids*, on the other hand, are those that the body can make, so they do not have to be obtained through the diet. Non-essential amino acids are not less essential than essential amino acids, but are given their name because the body has the ability to make them from other foods that we eat. The table below lists the different essential and non-essential amino acids.

Essential & Non-Essential Amino Acids

Essential Amino Acids		Non-Essential Amino Acids	
• Tryptophan	• Leucine	• Glycine	• Cystine
• Valine	• Lysine	• Arginine	• Proline
•Threonine	• Phenylalanine	• Glutamic Acid	• Aspartic Acid
• Isoleucine	• Methionine	• Glutamine	• Serine
	• Histidine	• Alanine	• Tyrosine
			• Asparagine

The task of memorizing the amino acids while trying to remember which are essential and which are non-essential has probably kept numerous students awake at night. A simple way to recall these facts is to assign a phrase to them that helps jog your memory. For example, consider the essential amino acids. Beginning with tryptophan and reading down the list, you may see that the first letter of each word spells the phrase "TV TILL PM." This memorable phrase may be used to recall the essential amino acids. Histidine, which is controversial due to debates about whether or not it is essential for adults, is usually left out of the list of essential amino acids. The same memory-jogging technique can be applied to the non-essential amino acids. Beginning with glycine and moving down the list yields the acronym "GAGG AC PASTA." Thus, the phrase "GAGG AC PASTA" provides one way for people to remember the non-essential amino acids.

An issue that often confuses people with regard to non-essential amino acids is that the classification *non-essential* gives the false impression that they serve no "essential" role. Ongoing research, however, is finding that nothing can be further from the truth. Studies reveal that individual non-essential amino acids may, in some circumstances, be essential. This has given rise to the term *conditionally essential amino acid*, which designates that, under some circumstances or conditions, an amino acid that normally is made in sufficient amounts might not be made efficiently enough to meet the body's needs. In such situations, supplementation may be needed. For instance, while glutamine is normally considered a non-essential amino acid, some research suggests that the body's need for glutamine may increase following surgery or disease.[66] Another example is histidine, which is essential in infants but may or may not be in adults. Some speculate that histidine may affect the immune system, although this point is controversial. Yet another example of a conditionally essential amino acid is arginine, as increased consumption may benefit people undergoing trauma such as surgery or severe burns.[67] For more on amino acids, please visit my website, Supplement-Geek.com.

Nitrogen Balance

The phrase *nitrogen balance* refers to a situation in which protein intake equals protein excretion or loss from the body. When protein intake equals protein loss, the body is said to be in a state of balance or homeostasis. A *positive nitrogen balance* occurs when protein intake exceeds protein excretion. Pregnant women, children, and those participating in a resistance training program all exhibit a positive nitrogen balance.[36] A *negative* nitrogen balance, on the other hand, occurs when protein excretion exceeds protein intake. This situation may occur when the body breaks down its own protein because of inadequate caloric intake. A negative nitrogen balance might be expected to occur in those suffering from long-term illness such as cancer or anorexia or in senior citizens who do not exercise or eat well. It is important to note that a negative nitrogen balance can occur even when protein intake is adequate or when it exceeds the recommended dietary allowance.[36] Inadequate caloric intake is the most important factor contributing to a negative nitrogen balance.

Protein & Weight Loss

Some people attempting to reduce body weight may choose to increase the amount of protein they consume. Science suggests that there may be some validity in this tactic. Because protein can stimulate the metabolism a bit, the addition of protein-containing meals to one's daily regimen might help foster weight loss. Protein also speeds water loss, which also helps reduce body weight, albeit temporarily. Given that dieting may increase protein breakdown, the addition of protein-rich foods to the diet may also spare body proteins from being catabolized. The calculation of how much protein is needed by adults will be addressed in a later chapter.

Macronutrient Determination

Sometimes the fitness professional may wish to show clients how to calculate the number of grams of carbohydrate, fat, and protein that are in his or her diet. This is helpful for those who do not wish to count calories but would rather focus on tracking grams of macronutrients consumed. For example, someone on a particular diet may be instructed to eat 190 grams of carbohydrates to maintain his or her dietary regimen. To illustrate this, let's use the following scenario. Suppose someone is following a diet consisting of 1,800 total calories per day with 60% of those calories coming from carbohydrates, 15% from protein, and 25% from fat. From these figures, one may determine the number of grams of carbohydrate, protein and fat that this diet provides.

Determine the number of grams of carbohydrate:
1,800 total calories X 0.6 = 1,080 calories from carbohydrates
1,080 ÷ 4 calories per gram = **270 grams of carbohydrates**

Determine the number of grams of protein:
1,800 total calories X 0.15 = 270 calories from protein
270 ÷ 4 calories per gram = **68 grams of protein**

Determine the number of grams of fat:
1,800 total calories x 0.25 = 450 calories from fat
450 ÷ 9 calories per gram = **50 g from fat**

Thus, this hypothetical 1,800-calorie diet consists of 270 grams of carbs, 68 grams of protein, and 50 grams of fat.

Some may wonder where the numbers 0.6, .15, and .25 originated. These are decimal equivalents of 60%, 15%, and 25% for carb, protein, and fat, respectively. Converting any number from a percent to a decimal is simply a matter of moving the decimal point two places to the left. For example, 60% equals 0.6.

Chapter 2

Energy & How We Make It

What Is Energy?

Energy is usually defined as the ability to do work. Work can be anything from reading these words to walking your dog, working out, or even keeping your heart beating--all activities require energy. We obtain energy from the foods that we eat, which contain the proteins, carbohydrates, and fats described in the last chapter. Let's now discuss how the body converts energy from food into the type of energy that it needs.

The Energy Contained in Food

The energy contained in food is measured in calories. A *calorie* is a unit of heat energy designating the amount of heat required to raise one kilogram (i.e., one liter) of water one degree Celsius. This definition gives rise to the alternative name for calories—*kilogram calories,* or *K calories* for short. Humans derive calories from the three macronutrients—protein, fat, and carbohydrate. As mentioned previously, the number of calories contained in each gram of protein, fat, and carbohydrate is known. While every gram of protein and carbohydrate contains 4 calories, every gram of fat contains 9. A concept seldom addressed, however, is that before these calories can be used, the body must first transform them into a usable type of energy. For all living things, including you and me, this form of energy is a molecule called ATP, which will now be discussed.

What Is ATP?

Humans, like all living things, must consume food to survive. Most people know that we use the energy contained in food to provide us with the energy needed to exercise and carry out daily activities. What some may not recognize is that the energy contained within food is not immediately available to us. In other words, the energy stored within the chemical bonds holding the atoms of food together must be rearranged into a form of energy that the body can use. For humans, that usable form of energy is stored in a molecule called *adenosine triphosphate* (ATP).

ATP is the ultimate energy molecule used to power all human activities. ATP consists of a molecule of adenosine chemically bonded to three phosphate atoms. There is a lot of energy contained within the chemical bond holding the third phosphate atom to the second phosphate atom, and when this chemical bond is broken, energy is released—this is the energy that we use.

What Does ATP Look Like?

The diagram below portrays an ATP molecule:

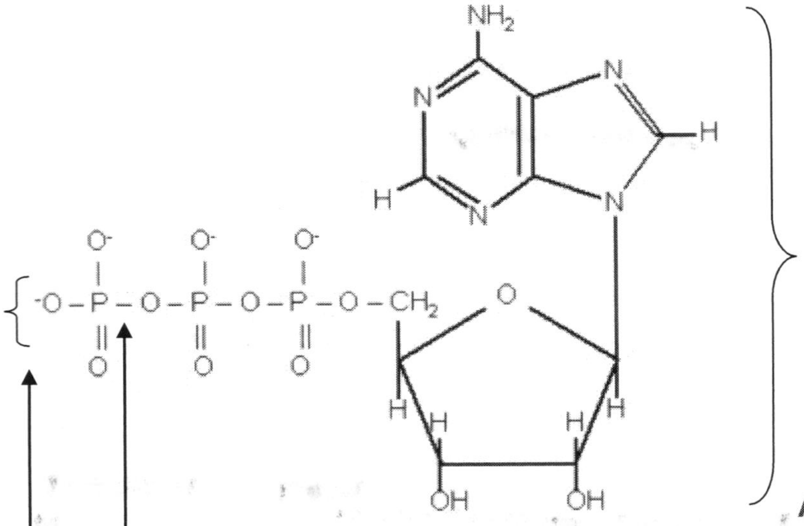

High-energy phosphate bond. When broken, much energy is released.

Three phosphate atoms

Adenosine

As can be seen in this picture, ATP is made of a molecule of adenosine (a type to sugar depicted on the right side of the picture) and three phosphate atoms (the three *P's* on the left side of the picture). The short lines between the phosphate atoms represent the energy-containing chemical bonds holding them together. The chemical bond attached to the last phosphate is called a *high-energy bond*, meaning that a large amount of energy is contained within it. When this chemical bond is broken, that energy is released to power human activities.

How Is ATP Made?

It should be understood that the human body has only enough ATP stored within it at any given time to power a few seconds of activity.[16] Consequently, ATP must be regenerated on a continual basis. The human body repeatedly produces ATP via the following chemical pathways: the *ATP/CP system*, *glycolysis*, and the *Krebs cycle*.

- **The ATP/CP System**. The ATP/CP system is an anaerobic energy pathway that consists of stored ATP and creatine phosphate (CP). Because both ATP and CP contain phosphate atoms, this system is sometimes referred to as *phosphagens*.

The limited amount of stored ATP breaks down first to power activity. During activities that require ATP to be regenerated at a faster rate than is normally possible, creatine phosphate is called into action. Creatine phosphate (CP) only comes into play during very short-lasting, highly intense physical activities such as sprinting or lifting very heavy weights. Acting as a supercharger for ATP production, creatine can help regenerate ATP for only a short period of approximately 30 seconds.[61] Thus, the creatine energy system is not used during low intensity activities such as walking, cycling, or other activities that can be carried out for long periods of time. Likewise, creatine does not come into play during relatively low intensity weight lifting plans such as circuit training or programs in which the resistance is lifted for 15 or more repetitions. Further information about creatine can be found in the dietary supplements chapter as well as on my website, Supplement-Geek.com.

More on ATP & CP

Some may be interested in learning the chemistry behind how ATP and CP work together. Below is a brief overview of this system.

The removal of the high-energy phosphate from ATP yields a molecule called adenosine diphosphate (ADP). The chemical reaction looks like this:

$$ATP \rightarrow ADP + P_i$$

P_i is the chemical symbol for an inorganic phosphate atom. Creatine phosphate can help reenergize ATP by donating its phosphate atom to ADP. The reaction looks like this:

$$CP + ADP \rightarrow ATP$$

After being regenerated, ATP once again breaks down, releasing its energy so that activity can continue.

- **Glycolysis.** Anaerobic glycolysis refers to a series of chemical reactions through which ATP (energy) is made via the anaerobic (no oxygen needed) breakdown of carbohydrates. Glycolysis is also known as the *lactic acid system*, a name which may lead individuals to mistakenly associate it with the burning muscles and muscle fatigue experienced during exercise. However, because the lactate that is actually produced through this process is not an acid, it does not play a role in exercise-induced muscle fatigue or muscle burning in and of itself.

The carbohydrate of choice used in glycolysis is *glucose*, which is sometimes referred to as blood sugar. When carbohydrates are eaten, they are chemically rearranged and transformed into the sugar glucose. Glucose, in turn, is stored in the body in the form of another molecule called *glycogen*. Remember that glycogen and glucose are very closely related. When glycogen is broken down, it releases glucose, which we can use to make energy.

What Is Aerobic Glycolysis?

It should come as little surprise that the human body is far more complex than many initially perceive. The process of glycolysis highlights this fact very well. Glycolysis is usually considered an anaerobic energy-generating pathway because oxygen is not needed for glycolysis to occur. Under some circumstances, however, glycolysis can be aerobic and use oxygen. This process is sometimes called *aerobic glycolysis*. which produces more ATP than its anaerobic counterpart. The downside of this is that ATP is not made as quickly.

Those struggling to understand which type of glycolysis—aerobic or anaerobic—occurs during different types of activities should remember that during high intensity activities during which ATP must be made rapidly, anaerobic glycolysis predominates. During low intensity activities during which ATP does not need to be made as quickly, on the other hand, aerobic glycolysis is more likely to occur.

- **The Krebs Cycle.** The *Krebs cycle* refers to a series of chemical reactions in which ATP is made from the breakdown of fat. The Krebs cycle is an aerobic pathway, meaning that it uses oxygen to metabolize fat. This process occurs in a specialized region of our cells called the **mitochondria**, within which fat-burning enzymes are located. During aerobic exercise training, mitochondria become larger and are produced in greater numbers, resulting in an improved ability to use fat for fuel. For this reason, aerobically-trained individuals use more fat and less glycogen even during sub-maximal exercise. Because the depletion of carbs (glycogen and glucose) can greatly hinder exercise performance, exercise-trained muscles that depend largely on fat for fuel have better endurance than weaker muscles that rely primarily on carbohydrates.

The Mitochondria

Mitochondria are often called "powerhouses of the cell" because the fat contained within them is energy-dense and capable of producing hundreds of ATP molecules. To better understand the way that mitochondria function, the analogy of a battery may be used. Those who have studied physics know that the batteries that power flashlights, CD players, cars, and more work by separating positive from negative electrical charges. When these electrical charges come together, energy is produced. In a similar way, mitochondria also separate positive and negative electrical charges, and when those electrical charges come together again, ATP is produced. Thus, mitochondria are essentially aerobic, rechargeable, fat-burning "batteries."

Another interesting fact about mitochondria is that when people regularly participate in aerobic exercise, mitochondria in the body's cells grow larger and multiply. Thus, a runner or cyclist would be expected to have more mitochondria in his or her cells than a sprinter or power lifter. Mitochondria are aerobic machines—when aerobic stress is regularly placed on the body during consistent exercise, the body sends a message to cells to step up production of mitochondria so that its needs may be met. The more mitochondria an athlete has, the more efficiently he or she burns fat.

People who don't work out regularly tend to have fewer mitochondria in their muscles. This is one reason why when novices start an exercise program, they have difficulty maintaining even "low" intensity of physical activity sometimes. Fitness trainers should remember this as they design training programs for their clients.

The different energy systems described in this chapter have been listed separately to facilitate the learning process. However, it should be kept in mind that they are all used simultaneously, albeit in varying degrees and circumstances, by the body. The intensity and duration of the activity being performed dictates whether a person is predominately making energy aerobically or anaerobically. If you are resting quietly while reading these words, the energy that your body is producing is roughly 60% aerobic and 40% anaerobic. As intensity of activity increases, however, the body begins to make energy more anaerobically because exercise of a greater intensity requires an increase in the rate of energy production. In such situations, pathways such as glycolysis and the ATP/CP system will likely be engaged.

Chapter 3

Macronutrient Use during Exercise

Although previously mentioned, the fact that all macronutrients are always being simultaneously used deserves further discussion. While all sources of calories—carbohydrate, fat, and protein—are utilized or burned for fuel at the same time, the ratio or relative contribution of each nutrient varies with exercise intensity and duration. During high intensity activities occurring over a short period of time, such as sprinting or heavy weight lifting, the body relies heavily upon carbohydrate and the breakdown of immediately-available ATP. As the duration of the exercise increases, a gradual shift occurs where fat breakdown begins to contribute significantly to exercise energy demands. Thus, a continuum of macronutrient utilization exists. At one end, anaerobic mechanisms (ATP and carbohydrate breakdown) provide the necessary energy for short bursts of high intensity exercise. At the other end of the continuum, aerobic metabolic processes (carbohydrate and fat breakdown) produce the energy to power longer low intensity workouts. For this reason, weight lifting is usually considered an anaerobic activity while walking and jogging are considered aerobic activities.

Exercise Intensity vs. Macronutrient Use	
Intensity/ Duration	Fuels Used
High Intensity, Short Lasting	ATP and Carbs
Low Intensity, Long Lasting	Carbs and Fats

Carbohydrates

Carbohydrates are the preferred fuel utilized during high intensity activity. As stated previously, the body relies more heavily upon carbohydrates as exercise intensity increases. Glycogen, the storage form of carbohydrate, is concentrated within the muscles and the liver. Within the muscles, gylcogen supplies large amounts of energy for the transitions from rest to moderate exercise and from moderate to intense exercise.[36] During moderate activity lasting at least 20 minutes, glycogen supplies between 40% and 50% of the body's energy demands, with the other half being supplied by fat.[36] Only small amounts of protein are used during moderate exercise. If exercise were to continue in the absence of any nutrient replenishment, glycogen levels would eventually fall below that needed to sustain exercise, resulting in fatigue and hindering exercise performance.

Another area where carbohydrates might help during exercise is by boosting the immune system. It is well-known that strenuous, long-duration aerobic activities like running marathons or triathlons can depress the immune system, resulting in a higher rate of colds and other illnesses developing in the days following the event. While the phenomenon is not yet fully understood, research suggests that carbohydrates consumed before and during prolonged high intensity aerobic exercise can support the immune system and may help reduce infections after an athletic event.[81]

Individuals should attempt to ingest the bulk of their carbohydrates in the form of complex carbohydrates such as fruits, vegetables, and whole grains. Complex carbohydrates are nutrient-dense foods, meaning that they contain a large number of nutrients relative to their weight and do not raise blood sugar as fast as simple, relatively nutrient-deficient carbohydrates such as candy, pies, cakes, and soda.

Glycogen vs. Glucose

A key concept often overlooked is that glucose and glycogen are different forms of the same molecule. Glucose, a simple carbohydrate, is often called blood sugar. Many glucose molecules chemically linked together form the complex carbohydrate called glycogen. When glycogen breaks down, it releases individual glucose molecules, which cells can then use to make energy (ATP). The relationship between glucose and glycogen is analogous to that of water and ice. Both water and ice are the same compound (H_2O) in different forms

---

Fat

Fat represents the major fuel source for light to moderate exercise. The abdominal region represents a particularly active area of fat mobilization, particularly when compared with fat stores located in the hip and thigh areas.[36] Again, as exercise intensity increases, there is a shift from fat to carbohydrate for fuel. With exercise training, a number of positive changes occur to facilitate the use of fat for fuel during exercise. These changes include:[36]

- increased rate of fat release from fat cells
- enhanced number of capillaries within trained muscles
- improved ability to transport fat through muscle cells
- improved ability to transport fat within muscle cells
- increased size and number of mitochondria
- enhanced quantity of fat-burning enzymes

Thus, exercise training (e.g., three or more months of walking or jogging) produces favorable metabolic changes that facilitate the use of fat as a fuel source during exercise.

Fat Breakdown during Exercise

A common misconception is that one must exercise aerobically for at least 20 minutes before fat is broken down for energy. In reality, fat breakdown begins to provide the body's energy needs after only a few minutes. Still, during longer durations of exercise, fat does begin to contribute more *significantly* to energy needs. For example, more fat is used to power the ATP/CP system after 20 minutes of exercise than after 5 minutes. Thus, a large percentage of fat is used as a fuel source during long sessions of low intensity exercise. This makes perfect sense when one considers that it takes time to shuttle fat from fat cells to the mitochondria and to break them down into smaller molecules to be burned for fuel.

There is an old saying that says, "Fat burns in a carbohydrate flame." This refers to the fact that fat breakdown depends in part on metabolic byproducts of carbohydrate metabolism that help during the fat-burning process. Reducing carbohydrates—as occurs through fasting or other low-carbohydrate diets—reduces the number of products from carbohydrate metabolic breakdown available to assist in the fat-burning process. This reduces fat breakdown and increases the body's production of molecules called *ketones*. Ketones are acidic molecules that, in excess, alter the acidity of the body and hinder its proper functioning.

Fat breakdown is also hindered when carbohydrate intake is inadequate to sustain long-lasting workouts. Runners and other endurance athletes sometimes refer to the depletion of carbohydrates during exercise as "hitting the wall."

The Skinny on the "Fat Burning" Program

Many people who have home exercise equipment or who belong to health clubs have probably noticed that many treadmills, ellipticals, and bikes feature a "Fat Burn" program. This program supposedly keeps people in the "fat burning zone" to foster weight loss. Let's look at the science behind this program to determine what role this type of workout might play in various exercise plans.

The basis of the fat burning program is that the body burns a greater percentage of fat at lower levels of exercise performed for long durations than during short, high intensity workouts. Let's take this reasoning and follow it to its ultimate conclusion. Suppose a person walks on a treadmill at 3 mph. Slowing the treadmill to 2 mph would cause the person's body to burn more fat because the intensity of the exercise is lower. Slowing the treadmill to 1 mph would burn even more fat. Now suppose that the person ceases exercise, sits down, and goes to sleep. Sleeping is actually the lowest intensity activity that any person can do. In fact, studies show that about 70% of the calories burned during sleep come from fat. The question, then, is why cannot people lose weight while sleeping if sleeping burns the most fat? The answer is simple—we don't burn many calories while sleeping, and the number of calories burned, not the amount of fat burned, that provides the key to weight loss. Thus, exercise fosters weight loss far more than sleeping.

The fat burning program does have its place, especially in exercise plans designed for untrained individuals not accustomed to working out. Such programs encourage the individual to maintain a relatively low intensity (usually around 60% of estimated max heart rate), which makes injury less likely and allows the person to perform the activity for a longer period of time to increase the total number of calories burned. Depending on the person's initial fitness level, he or she may adapt to the fat burning program after a few months. From that point forward, they may opt for the "cardio program" found on many pieces of cardiovascular exercise equipment. The cardio program encourages people to exercise at a slightly higher intensity (about 80% of maximal heart rate) than the fat burning program.

Protein

As stated before, protein forms thousands of complex molecules in the body. Since protein is crucial to health, it makes sense that it does not provide the bulk of the body's energy requirements at rest or during exercise. Contributing only 2–10% of the energy needed for physical activity, protein supplies far less fuel than either carbohydrates or fat and is not ideal for powering an individual through a workout.[24] This is especially true in individuals who have consumed an adequate amount of carbohydrate, as carbs reduce protein breakdown during exercise. In those who have less than optimal carbohydrate and calorie intakes, on the other hand, protein is broken down in greater amounts.[45] Over time, this may slow muscle growth and hinder exercise performance.

Older adults individuals with eating disorders, and those with other serious medical issues may not consume enough protein to meet daily energy needs. This chronic lack of protein can lead to sarcopenia and other forms of muscle wasting. In such instances, it is recommended that the personal trainer refer to person to a registered dietitian who can work closely with the individual to identify the appropriate course of action for long-term health.

Chapter 4

Nutrition and Exercise

This chapter addresses the types and amounts of major nutrients thought to cultivate optimal exercise capacity.

Carbohydrate

Exercise places a demand on the body that requires steady, relatively fast energy production. Because it is relatively easy for the body to draw energy from carbohydrates, they represent the primary macronutrient used during exercise. This is especially true during high intensity, short periods of activity such as resistance training. During exercises such as cycling and marathon running, carbohydrates are often referred to as the *rate-limiting nutrient*. This phrase reflects the importance of carbohydrates for the continuation of exercise. In other words, when carbohydrate reserves are depleted, the body can no longer perform activities efficiently. Research demonstrates that the human body has approximately 1,200–1,500 calories in the form of glycogen (the storage form of carbohydrates), enough energy to run non-stop for about 20 miles.[36] Because marathons, century bike rides, triathlons, and other similar athletic events usually last longer than 20 miles, endurance athletes are often seen eating during events. If they do not eat, glycogen reserves will eventually be depleted, resulting in subpar exercise performance.

Because carbohydrates are essential for optimal exercise performance, they are often recommended in high amounts for athletes. One seldom-mentioned function of carbohydrates is that they help reduce protein breakdown. Thus, carbs help spare muscle protein (and other proteins) from being consumed for fuel.

In general, carbohydrates should contribute between 55 and 65% of total calorie intake and should be derived from nutrient-dense complex carbohydrates such as fruits, vegetables, and unprocessed grains. Again, complex carbs are stressed over simple carbs because of their higher nutrient and water content. Moreover, complex carbohydrates do not typically cause an immediate spike in blood glucose levels as simple sugars do. Such a rapid elevation in blood glucose can result in the quick release of the hormone insulin, which drastically lowers blood sugar and stimulates appetite. This, in turn, may cause lethargy and less-than-optimal performance during exercise.

Where Do the Extra Carbs Go?

As mentioned previously, the body stores roughly 1,200–1,500 calories in the form of glycogen. Some readers may wonder what happens to carbs eaten after the body has reached its carbohydrate storage capacity. The answer is simple: the body converts the extra carbs to fat and stores them in the body. Thus, even though eating carbs is healthy, eating extra calories in the form carbohydrates can lead to weight gain in the form of fat.

The Glycemic Index

Because not all carbohydrates are processed the same way, simply calling sugars "simple" or "complex" may not give us the whole picture. Instead, the glycemic index may provide a more complete picture of the sugars contained in various foods.

The glycemic index (GI) is a 0–100 rating scale that shows how quickly an ingested carbohydrate elevates blood sugar levels. The higher the number, the faster the carbohydrate raises blood sugar. Glucose and white bread are often used as reference points and given ratings of 100, indicating that they raise blood sugar extremely rapidly. A food with a glycemic index of 70, for example, raises blood sugar levels 70% as quickly as the same amount of glucose or white bread would.[42]

Some have argued that eating foods with low glycemic indices is superior to eating foods with high glycemic indices. For example, low-glycemic foods tend to help people feel fuller longer and might not stimulate appetite as significantly as foods with a high glycemic index. Some evidence suggests that a low-glycemic diet may stave off type II diabetes and other diseases as well. However, determining the glycemic index of a given food can be difficult, as each of the following factors may affect this measurement:[44]

- Is the food cooked or raw?
- What is the fiber content of the food?
- How ripe is the food (ripe banana vs. non-ripe, for example)?
- What is the portion size (8 oz vs. 12 oz of a food, for example)?
- Is the food being eaten with other foods? If so, then the foods together may have a different GI than either food would alone.

Foods with a rating of 70 or more are considered high on the glycemic index, foods with a GI of 56–69 are regarded as moderate glycemic index, and foods with a GI of less than 55 are usually thought of as low-glycemic. Foods such as meats, which contain no carbohydrates, do not have a glycemic index, while those containing a large amount of fat may actually have a low glycemic index, but because of their fat content, they may contain a significant number of calories. Thus, "low-calorie" and "low-GI" do not always mean the same thing.

Fruits and vegetables tend to be low on the glycemic index and, from a nutrition standpoint, they tend to offer more vitamins, minerals, and fiber than foods higher on the index. Thus, fruits and vegetables figure prominently in glycemic index eating plans. The table below organizes several different foods according to their glycemic index.

Glycemic Index of Foods		
Low GI (55 or less)	Medium GI (55-69)	High GI (70 or above)
• Milk	• Rye bread	• White bread
• Yogurt	• Sodas	• French fries
• Banana	• Pineapple	• Corn Flakes™ cereal
• All Bran™ cereal	• Brown rice (steamed)	• Bran Flakes™ cereal
• Grapes	• White rice (Uncle Ben's,™ boiled)	• Cheerios™ cereal
• Pure Protein™ bar (strawberry shortcake)	• Met-Rx® meal replacement drink (Vanilla)	• Clif bar® (cookies and cream)
• Soy milk	• Pizza (cheese)	• Boiled potatoes
• Sweet potatoes	• Oatmeal cookies	• Baked potatoes
• Nuts	• Ice cream (vanilla & chocolate)	• Jelly beans
• Baked beans	• Angel food cake	• Coco Pops™ cereal

Adapted from glycemicindex.com

Glycemic Index & Exercise: Practical Uses

Currently, the role of the glycemic index and its implications for exercise performance remains controversial.[42, 45] That being said, the glycemic index can be utilized in some practical ways by athletes desiring to maximize performance. Exercise, especially in its aerobic form, depletes glycogen levels. This reduction in glycogen is accompanied by an increase in the enzyme called *glycogen synthase*, which makes glycogen to replace what has been used. Following exercise, humans have a window of opportunity of about 30–60 minutes within which the body is most capable of replenishing glycogen reserves. This is why it is often recommended that athletes eat as soon as possible after exercise. If the tactic of eating within 30–60 minutes after exercise were to be combined with eating a high-glycemic food, the result might equal greater-than-normal glycogen storage.[69] This, in turn, might benefit athletes involved in daily bouts of long-duration exercise such as cycling in the Tour de France, participating the Olympic Games, or engaging in comparable grueling athletic events. Moreover, those following strength training programs might eat some protein along with a high-glycemic food in order to enhance the body's uptake of amino acids needed to rebuild muscle.

During long-lasting activities such as running marathons, athletes traditionally eat carbohydrates to sustain blood sugar levels and to prevent glycogen depletion. The consumption of high-glycemic foods during such endurance events might decrease exercise performance by causing a large spike in insulin and a drastic reduction in blood sugar. In contrast, low- to moderate-glycemic foods, which do not dramatically increase insulin, may be a better choice during exercise. For this reason, marathon runners and other endurance athletes frequently eat bananas, a classic low-glycemic food, during events.

Glycemic Index and Weight Loss

Some have argued that emphasizing the glycemic index when choosing foods to eat can promote weight loss. Unfortunately, there is little scholarly agreement when it comes to determining whether or not this is true. Many fruits and vegetables, which are recommended for those desiring to shed excess weight, are low-glycemic foods. However, most evidence to date suggests that the reduced calorie consumption associated with eating these foods— not their place on the glycemic index— is the most important factor for weight loss.

The Glycemic Load

The concept of glycemic load is an extension of the glycemic index. Remember that the glycemic index can be affected by the amount of food eaten, which makes a diet based on the glycemic index rather difficult to follow. The glycemic load (GL) may, according to some researchers, offer a better guideline for eating well.

The glycemic load is defined as the glycemic index of a food multiplied by the number of grams of carbohydrate. The resulting number is then divided by 100.[71] Research finds that people who eat a diet with a high glycemic load tend to suffer from more diseases such as diabetes.[71] Diets with relatively high glycemic loads diets may also be linked to elevated C reactive protein (CRP) levels, which may play a role in the development of heart disease.[71] Foods such as fruits and vegetables, grains, and beans tend to have a low glycemic load as well as a low glycemic index, making them important components of a nutritious eating plan.

The Glycemic Load	
GL Range	**Meaning**
≤ 10	Low GL
11 to 19	Medium GL
≥ 20	High GL

Glycemic Index & Glycemic Load of Select Foods			
Food	Amount	Glycemic Index	Glycemic Load
Baked potatoes	1 medium	85	26
Jelly beans	1 oz	78	22
White rice	1 cup	64	23
Brown rice	1 cup	55	18
Orange	1 medium	42	5
All Bran™ cereal	1 cup	38	9
Cornflakes	1 cup	81	21
Skim milk	1 cup	32	4

Deciphering glycemic index and glycemic load can be a challenge. The table below shows how the different scales compare with each other:

Glycemic Index vs. Glycemic Load: How they Compare		
	GI Range	GL Range
Low	< 55	<10
Medium	55 to 69	11 to 19
High	≥ 70	≥ 20

Interesting evidence exists that links low glycemic index and low glycemic load diets to reduced disease risk. Remember that both measurements emphasize the value of complex carbohydrates, fruits, vegetables, grains, and beans. For the most part, this remains consistent with popular dietary recommendations such as those advocated by the Academy of Nutrition and Dietetics. Thus, people eating healthy diets consisting of grains, vegetables, fruits, and legumes may already adhere to recommendations made according to the low glycemic index and low glycemic load philosophies. Remembering this fact may help people avoid confusion and focus on continuing to eat a nutritious diet featuring plenty of produce and whole foods even as research on the glycemic index and the glycemic load develops.

Protein

Most of the energy used during exercise comes from carbohydrates and fat, while protein contributes little fuel for physical activity. The Recommended Dietary Allowance (RDA) for protein for non-exercising individuals is 0.8 grams per kilogram of body weight (kg/BW), or 0.36 grams per pound.[134] Thus, protein intake depends partially on how much a person weighs. For example, a person weighing 150 lbs (68 kg) has a protein RDA of 68 kg X 0.8 = 55.5 grams, or about two ounces of protein. A person who weighs 200 lbs, on the other hand, has an RDA of about 73 grams of protein. Other factors also play affect an individual's protein requirements, including age, medical status, pregnancy, protein quality (animal vs. plant), total calorie intake, workout experience (beginner vs. trained), exercise intensity, and exercise duration. While studies find that the recommendation of 0.8 grams/kilogram is sufficient for most young, healthy individuals,[36] other recommendations call for slightly higher amounts of protein for those who exercise regularly or intensely.[30,134,142]

Goal	Amount (g/kg)	Amount (g/lb)
RDA	0.8	0.36
Weekend warrior	1.1 to 1.4	0.5 to 0.6
Aerobic athlete	1.2 to 2	0.5 to 0.9
Weight lifter	1.4 to 2	0.6 to 0.9

Note: kg=kilogram. 1 kilogram = 2.2 pounds.

Notice that there is no standard agreement about how much protein is best for all people. This reinforces the fact that protein recommendations must be individualized according to many factors, including but not limited to those mentioned above. Notice also that the upper limit for both aerobic exercise and weight lifting is usually set at 0.9 grams. Many trainers round up to 1.0, giving the all-too-common answer of "1 gram per pound" when clients inquire about how much protein they need. As can be seen from the table, this is not always the correct answer and, in some cases, may be notably too high. Additionally, keep in mind that the protein recommendations presented here are not rigid regulations, but are offered as general guidelines to help fitness professionals provide responsible answers to their clients' questions regarding protein.

It is often stated by nutrition professionals that the average non-exercising American exceeds the RDA for protein.[36] To illustrate, some research has noted that US men age 20 and over consume 152% of the RDA for protein, while women consume 127%.[78] As stated previously, protein is not the fuel of choice during exercise and is not typically used in large quantities during athletic events. Rather, carbohydrate and fat contribute greater amounts of energy during periods of physical activity. While the ideal amount of protein necessary for optimal exercise performance is not currently known, some research suggests that for most people, that amount is probably within the 1.2–1.8 g/kg BW range.[134]

The branched-chain amino acids (leucine, isoleucine, and valine) are used for fuel during physical activity and are sometimes supplemented by those looking to improve exercise capacity. Some research suggests that the branched-chain amino acids (BCAAs) limit the entry of the amino acid called tryptophan into the brain. Given that tryptophan helps make serotonin, a neurochemical that plays a role in sleep, adding BCAAs to the diet may lower serotonin levels and thus extend the time it takes to experience fatigue. This intriguing theory is also a controversial one, as studies to date have been unable to show conclusively that ingestion of branched-chain amino acids during exercise enhances athletic performance.[32] If BCAAs work, they might be best-suited for professional athletes and for those participating in endurance events such as marathons and long-range cycling events. Of the BCAAs, **leucine** often receives the most attention because it appears to play a role in the synthesis of muscle protein after exercise.[142] Some research suggests that a "leucine threshold" needs to be achieved to kick start the muscle protein synthesis process. Research suggests that this threshold may be between 1-3 grams per day.

When people discuss protein, they often wonder whether it is best to eat it before or after exercise. While both strategies work, some evidence supports the notion that eating protein immediately (i.e., within 1 hour) after exercise is superior to eating it prior to exercise.[134] That said, other research hints that timing meals may not be needed. No matter who is right, meal timing is probably most critical for older adults, professional athletes or those with wasting diseases.

Combining protein with a carbohydrate is better than protein alone, given that carbs stimulate insulin production, which helps with the assimilation of amino acids. Another factor that needs to be taken into account when choosing post-workout foods is that essential amino acids are better than non-essential varieties at stimulating muscle protein synthesis.

Another question that often arises with respect to protein is how much can be absorbed from one meal. Many people reading these words have probably heard that people can only absorb 35–40 grams of protein per meal, but in reality, there is no solid proof for this. The body efficiently absorbs the protein from most of what you eat throughout the day. That said, most people can be served well by aiming for between 20-25 grams per meal if they are working out.

High-protein Diets & Weight Loss

Some people attempting to lose weight opt to increase the amount of protein in their diet by consuming more protein-containing foods or more high-protein shakes, food bars, or other supplements. Protein may be an effective aid for accomplishing weight-loss goals for a few reasons. First, protein, which contains roughly 4 calories per gram, is relatively low in calories. Eating protein at the expense of other high-calorie foods such as those containing a large amount of fat can create a calorie deficit that fosters weight loss. Second, protein tends to help people feel satiated for a longer period of time than carbohydrates. Thus, people who emphasize protein in the diet may not feel hungry as often and may not ingest as many calories as those who opt for carbohydrate-rich foods. Third, protein has a mild thermogenic effect. The *thermic effect of food* (TEF) relates to how much energy the body must invest to metabolize (i.e., digest, process, transport, etc.) the food in question. Some estimates identify the thermic effect of protein as 30% greater than fat, whose low TEF makes it the most easily assimilated macronutrient). Thus, high-protein diets may slightly and temporarily elevate metabolism to increase the number of calories burned over time. Fourth, protein promotes the loss of water from the body. When protein is metabolized, it makes a compound called urea, which is flushed from the body in the urine, using water in the process. This dehydrating property of protein is sometimes used by bodybuilders to promote a more vascular appearance.

How Protein Might Help Weight Loss
1. Protein is low in calories
2. Protein slows digestion
3. Protein boosts metabolism
4. Protein promotes water loss

While protein can play a beneficial role in helping people lose weight, emphasizing protein at the expense of other healthy foods is not a sensible approach to weight loss. The most effective strategy for weight reduction is reducing the number of calories eaten. One particularly noteworthy drawback to high-protein diets is that they are not ideal for people who exercise regularly. Because the body relies on carbohydrates and fat to power most activities, increasing protein consumption may negatively influence energy levels and hinder athletic performance. Thus, people on high-protein diets (at the expense of carbs and/or fat) must be prepared for the possibility that their athletic performance and endurance in the gym may decrease.

Are Protein Supplements Needed?

It is often said that a healthy diet provides all of the protein that the body needs build muscle and function properly. While this is, indeed, true, some people may find it easier and more efficient to add a protein bar or protein shake to their diet to insure that they consume the amount of protein that they need. A vast array of protein supplements is available (and more options are added to the market all the time) to accommodate the needs of busy consumers. Like all supplements, protein bars, shakes, and other products are designed to *supplement* the diet, not to *replace* real food. Still, research does suggest that protein supplements can contribute to muscle growth, and high-quality supplements are suspected to be as profitable as protein-containing foods for this purpose.

The primary advantage of protein supplements is their convenience. While this can be an asset to those with busy schedules, quality protein supplements may also benefit those who have trouble eating, including seniors. Older adults usually do not eat as much as they should and may have trouble chewing because of dentures. Inadequate levels of dietary protein could cause the body to cannibalize the protein reserves found in the muscles. In such instances, the addition of a quality protein supplement to the diet may help seniors to preserve lean muscle mass. The safeguarding of muscle mass as one grows older can have a profound positive influence on the quality (and duration) of life by keeping muscles strong and by offsetting sarcopenia (age-related muscle loss). Additional protein might also boost the immune system and promote the proper functioning of vital organs. When discussing protein with seniors and other with special dietary needs, the fitness professional must also remember that, though protein is a crucial nutrient, too much might actually enhance bone loss. Thus, the protein intake of older adults should be monitored closely.

Ultimately, the decision to use a protein supplement is an individual one. Before deciding on a protein supplement for a client, the fitness professional should first determine how much protein (and calories) the individual currently consumes. This can be accomplished by having the client fill out a three-day food journal or by using free websites or applications. After the daily nutritional profile has been outlined, the fitness professional can weigh the information obtained against factors such as the frequency and intensity of exercise, the client's goals, and whether or not those goals are being achieved. Keep in mind that the number of calories, amount of protein, and levels of saturated fat and other nutrients can vary greatly from product to product. Also remember that not all protein supplements are appropriate for everyone. Health problems can also influence protein needs. For clients with significant health issues, its recommended referring them to a registered dietitian. For more information on protein and other supplements, see my website, Supplement-Geek.com.

Can We Eat Too Much Protein?

A common question that often arises when discussing protein is whether it is possible to consume too much of the macronutrient. The short answer to this is yes—of course this is possible, especially if protein emphasized at the expense of other nutritious foods. Most people, however, are truly asking whether there is a threshold of protein past which side effects may begin to appear. Most experts stipulate that no more than 2 grams of protein per kilogram of body weight be consumed. The most frequently-cited reason for this are that excess protein can place undue stress on kidneys, causing kidney problems. One review of literature concerning this issue, however, found that high-protein diets (defined as 1.5 grams per kilogram of body weight) do not appear to harm the kidneys of healthy adults.[72] More research must be conducted to verify these conclusions and to conclusively determine whether or not high-protein diets negatively impact the function of healthy adult kidneys. Because many professional athletes commonly use more than 2–2.5 grams of protein per kilogram of body weight, some might contend that high-protein diets are less risky than originally thought. However, professional athletes tend to be in better overall health than the average individual, making it difficult to use this data to draw conclusions about the general public. Furthermore, high-protein intakes are certainly not appropriate for those who have liver or kidney problems or other medical disorders. Thus, optimal protein intake must be determined on a case-by-case basis.

Another widely discussed potential side effect of high-protein diets concerns its effect on bones. Specifically, protein is known to leach calcium from the bones. Some speculate that high-protein diets may be a risk factor for osteoporosis, but research does not universally support this theory.[134] When examining this question, it is interesting to consider those who consume the large quantities of protein, including athletes such as bodybuilders and power lifters. Generally, osteoporosis is not a problem for these individuals. Is it possible that any deleterious effects of protein on bones might be offset by the positive effects of resistance training? This is an interesting theory worthy of further study.

Protein and Vegetarians

Some people choose to consume a diet composed of only fruits and vegetables. The fitness professional should have a general understanding of the nuances of vegetarianism and its influence on exercise and exercise performance. People have a variety of motives behind their choice to become a vegetarian, including religious, health, and ethical reasons. Research finds vegetarianism is associated with numerous health benefits, including a reduced risk of a variety of diseases. Within the lifestyle of vegetarianism, several subgroups exist:[12]

- **Lacto-ovo-vegetarians**: eat vegetables, milk, and eggs but not meat or seafood.

- **Lacto-vegetarian**: consume vegetables, milk, and milk products but not eggs.

- **Ovo-vegetarians**: consume vegetables and eggs but not milk or milk products.

- **Fruitarians**: consume only fruits and nuts.

As stated in previous sections, some amino acids are essential and must be obtained from the diet (or through supplements). Foods such as meat, fish, and poultry that contain all of the essential amino acids in the necessary amounts are called *complete proteins*. Because essential amino acids tend to be scarcer in vegetables than they are in meats, vegetables are usually referred to as *incomplete proteins*. However, the decision to become a vegetarian does not preclude one from building muscle or competing athletically. While many foods that vegetarians consume are incomplete proteins when eaten alone, they can be combined with other foods to make complete protein sources. For example, the following foods, when combined together, will result in a complete, high-quality protein capable of fostering muscle growth:[30]

- Rice and beans
- Corn and beans
- Corn and lima beans
- Pasta and bean soup

Another important thing to remember is that the above foods do not have to be eaten in the same meal to be effective. Consuming complementary incomplete proteins within 24 hours of each other is just as effective as eating them simultaneously.[12] Thus, avoiding meat does not prevent one from eating healthfully. In fact, on some levels, vegetarians are healthier than those whose diet consists primarily of beef and other meat products in that they tend to develop less obesity, cancer, diabetes, and heart disease than meat eaters.

Another option for vegetarians is to eat soy. While derived from plants, soy is a complete protein and is therefore a viable alternative for those who do not consume meat. Studies show that diets containing 25–50 grams of soy per day can also help lower cholesterol levels.

One possible drawback to a strict non-animal containing diet is that vegetarians may be deficient in some vitamins and minerals, specifically vitamin B_{12}, iron, and zinc.[30] These deficiencies, however, can be easily alleviated by taking a daily multivitamin containing the RDA for all vitamins and minerals.

Fat

Contrary to popular belief, fat is not a useless or unhealthy macronutrient. Fat provides the abundance of the body's energy needs during exercise. Examples of activities that use fat as a fuel source include walking, swimming, biking, hiking, and bicycling. Comparatively, little fat is utilized for fuel during resistance training programs. In the past, media has portrayed fat as an undesirable nutrient, but the fitness professional must recognize that fat is a valuable asset for those involved in exercise training. Because fat is an energy-dense nutrient (i.e., it contains 9 calories per gram), it is much easier to use fat rather than protein or carbohydrates to add calories needed to maintain body weight and muscle mass during exercise programs. In addition, some evidence suggests that the normal (and necessary) rise in testosterone that occurs following resistance training is decreased in those who consume a low fat diet.[58]

Fat comes in three different forms: *monounsaturated fat*, *polyunsaturated fat,* and *saturated fat.* From a health standpoint, mono- and polyunsaturated fats tend to better for us. Diets high in saturated fats, on the other hand, have been shown to raise the risk of heart disease. From a calorie standpoint, however, all types of fat have 9 calories per gram. This is important to remember because it is possible to gain weight even when following a diet high in healthy fats. Remember, calories are the key to weight loss (and weight gain)—not fat.

Current recommendations for this macronutrient advocate that no more than 30% of total daily calorie intake should be derived from fats, with the majority of this amount coming from unsaturated fats. Some diets may advocate lower amounts, but fat is necessary because it not only makes food taste better and helps satiate the appetite. Thus, diets lower than 30% fat may be more difficult to maintain for an extended period of time.

High-Fat Diets and Exercise Performance

Since fat provides a wealth of energy during exercise, some may wonder whether eating a high fat can boost exercise performance. The answer to this question appears to be no. When athletes are placed on diets containing various amounts of fat, those higher in fat do not appear to improve exercise performance.[69]

Trans Fats

As saturated fats began to fall out of public favor, some companies began using partially hydrogenated fats as an alternative to fully hydrogenated varieties. Partially hydrogenated fats are less saturated than saturated fats and were once thought to be a healthier alternative. Research, however, shows that during the process of making partially hydrogenated fats, trans fats are created. Because of this, trans fatty acids are sometimes found in products that contain saturated fats, such as baked goods and fast food. Trans fats are on the "radar screens" of many nutritionists because they appear to decrease HDL and increase LDL.

By lowering HDL and increasing LDL, trans fats have the potential to clog arteries and elevate heart disease risk. Because of this, the FDA mandates that food labels explicitly list trans fats. Foods with less than 0.5 grams of trans fats per serving can still say they have "0" trans fats. However, "per serving" is the essential aspect of this statement. If a package of "trans fat free food" containing 10 servings is eaten in its entirety, then approximately 5 grams of trans fats (0.5 x 10) may have been consumed. Given current concerns about nutrition and its influence on long-term health, this label loophole will likely be corrected in the near future.

Chapter 5

Boosting Exercise Performance

Both professional athletes and weekend warrior are consistently trying different ways to improve their exercise performance and accelerate the speed with which they adapt to exercise. This chapter reviews some of the most popular methods currently used to achieve these goals and fosters a working understanding of which strategies may be most effective.

Carbohydrate Loading

This method of boosting exercise performance has been used by triathletes and other ulta-endurance athletes for years. Technically called *glycogen super-compensation*, carbohydrate loading (or simply, "carbo loading"), takes advantage of the body's enhanced ability to store carbohydrate (glycogen) after a period of carbohydrate restriction. The action of restricting carbs causes the body to increase its output of *glycogen synthase*, an enzyme that helps make glycogen. An increase in this enzyme may help the body load up on glycogen when carbs are reintroduced into the diet.

While a number of "recipes" to achieve this glycogen-loading effect exist, some strategies are more common than others. Typically, an athlete participates in aerobic exercise for approximately 7–10 days prior to a competition in order to purposely exhaust his or her glycogen reserves. This is activity is accompanied by a conscious decision to restrict the consumption of carbohydrates. Sometimes only 100 grams of carbohydrates per day are eaten! This is an extremely low quantity that is almost certain to drastically decrease an individual's exercise ability. Approximately three to four days before the event, the athlete then eats a high-carbohydrate diet (upwards of 400–700 grams of carbs per day). Research finds that carbo-loading has the potential to cause a 50%–100% increase in the amount of glycogen stored. For those who do not wish to do any math when carbo-loading, another version of the method calls for the person to simply increase carbohydrate intake while cutting back on the volume of exercise performed.

Studies show that carbo-loading seems to work best for aerobic endurance events lasting more than 90 minutes.[36] It is presumably less effective for those who take part in 5K runs or who workout a few days a week at the gym. To determine whether carbo-loading improves exercise performance for those who strength train, further study is required.[30]

A word of caution for those considering carbo-loading: The body will eventually adapt to it, making it less effective. Thus, this technique is not something to implement on a regular basis. In addition, it is probably wise to experiment with carbo-loading before the actual athletic event. That way, the individual can determine how he or she reacts to the practice prior to the day of the competition.

Caffeine Supplementation

Caffeine, a stimulant found in coffee, caffeinated sodas, and some pre-workout supplements, is often used by athletes to boost mental alertness, improve reaction time, and enhance overall exercise performance. Studies show that caffeine can:

1. promote the release of adrenaline (epinephrine), a stimulating hormone, from the adrenal glands
2. stimulate the release of calcium from cells, which in turn helps promote muscle contraction
3. prompt the release of fatty acids into the blood, where they can be burned for fuel
4. heighten overall psychological and physiological arousal to improve reaction time and exercise performance

Most evidence of caffeine's ability to improve exercise performance stems from studies of long duration aerobic events like marathons. Findings regarding caffeine's effects on the quality of short, high intensity events such as sprinting, on the other hand, are mixed. While some studies suggest that the stimulant may aid exercise performance, others hint that it does not. Generally, these studies use between 2 and 10 mg/kg of caffeine. Ultimately, the effect of caffeine on exercise performance probably varies from person to person, and habitual use of caffeine may alter its effectiveness.

It should be noted that, while commonly used by millions of people around the world, caffeine is not without risks. Doses of over 200 mg a day may speed heart rate and interfere with sleeping, while doses above 10 grams of caffeine a day (150 mg/kg) can be fatal. Competitive athletes should remember that high doses of caffeine are illegal in the Olympics.

Caffeine, along with other stimulants, forms the backbone for many pre-workout drinks. Most of these products are inadequately supported with proof that they actually improve exercise performance. Without solid evidence, it may be wise to assume that such products are essentially expensive caffeine supplements.

Water

As important as protein, fat, carbohydrate, vitamins, and minerals are to the maintenance of health and exercise performance, water is equally as important. This becomes particularly apparent when one considers that the average person can usually last for months without food, yet will die after just a week without water. Based on this fact alone, water may even be considered the most important nutrient of all. Depending on age, gender, and body composition, water comprises between 40% and 70% of body mass.[36] With respect to muscle and fat, water comprises 65–75% and 50%, respectively.[36]

Functions of Water

Water serves a variety of purposes in the body:

- Water helps transport nutrients and gasses throughout the body.
- Water serves as a medium for a vast array of chemical reactions.
- Water helps lubricate joints.
- Water helps dissipate excess heat, thus helping maintain a consistent body temperature.

Consequences of Dehydration

Dehydration refers to a situation when fluid intake does not match fluid loss.[36] Almost all physical exertion results in some fluid loss. For example, a moderate, one-hour exercise session can result in a loss of between 0.5 and 1.5 liters of sweat.[36] Higher intensity exercise, especially in a hot environment, increases fluid loss even more. Studies show that a fluid loss of only 2% of body weight can significantly decrease exercise performance.[21]

The average person consumes approximately 91 ounces of water each day.[36] Since fluid loss via perspiration can increase dramatically during times of physical activity, fluid intake must increase to as much as 6 times the normal requirement during these periods. During exercise in high heat and humidity, fluid loss may exceed ten pounds, and fluid intake must increase even more.[32]

How Water Is Lost From the Body

There are essentially four ways that water is lost from the body:

1. Water loss through the skin. This form of water loss, which occurs when water is lost from the sweat glands, helps the body to cool itself. The small amount of constant sweat through which the body consistently cools itself is called *insensible perspiration.*

2. Water loss as water vapor. This represents water that is lost when we exhale.

3. Water loss from urine. The average loss of water from urine is approximately 1.5 quarts per day.

4. Water loss in feces. Surprisingly enough, water makes up about 70% of fecal matter.[36] The loss of fluid though the feces can increase dramatically during bouts with diarrhea.

Fluid Intake and Exercise

Prior to exercise, individuals should be well-hydrated, so fluid intake should begin before exercise even begins. This is especially true for cyclists, triathletes, and other athletes competing in lengthy endurance events. A quick way to check for ample hydration is to observe the color of urine. Dark yellow urine that has a strong odor may indicate less-than-adequate hydration.[36] Fluid hydration recommendations call for individuals to drink approximately 17–20 ounces 2–3 hours before exercise and approximately 7–10 ounces of fluid 10–20 minutes before exercise.[15] This should allow ample time for the fluid to hydrate the body in preparation for physical activity. During exercise, individuals should consume 7–10 ounces every 10–20 minutes for the duration of the event. Following exercise, it is not uncommon to lose weight via fluid loss from sweat. To determine if weight loss has occurred following exercise, individuals should weigh themselves before and after physical activity. New recommendations on fluid replacement following exercise call for the ingestion of 3 cups (24 ounces) of fluid for every pound of fluid lost during exercise.[15] Ideally, this fluid should be consumed within 2 hours following exercise.[15] Properly scheduling fluid replacement before, during, and after exercise will ensure that circulation and sweating function at optimal levels.

Fluids: Before, During and After Exercise

Time	Fluid Intake
• 10–20 before exercise	7–10 oz
• During exercise	7–10 oz every 10–20 min
• After exercise	24 oz per pound lost

Alcohol

Alcohol is a poor substitute for water during athletic events because it dehydrates the body and impairs exercise performance. Alcohol is a depressant to the nervous system, which further reduces athletic performance by decreasing balance and coordination. Because alcohol is a diuretic, it speeds the loss of water, vitamins, and minerals, including thiamin, vitamin B_6, and calcium.[30] In addition to being devoid of significant vitamins, minerals, or other nutrients, alcohol is also a potent source of calories, with every gram of alcohol containing 7 calories. That is almost as many calories as are contained in fat (9 calories/ gram). While evidence does exist to show that moderate alcohol consumption may elevate HDL levels, so, too, does exercise. Excessive alcohol consumption can raise blood pressure and elevate triglyceride levels and may even reduce glycogen re-storage and testosterone production.[30]

Sports Drinks

Some may opt to drink beverages such as sports drinks rather than water. Consuming such drinks may actually be beneficial simply because their appealing flavor encourages consumers to consume more fluid. One study compared the level of voluntary fluid intake among plain water, grape-flavored water, and grape-flavored water containing 6% carbohydrate and salts (electrolytes).[35] This study found that the beverage containing the carbohydrates and salts resulted in the greatest volume of fluid ingested.

Another advantage of sports drinks becomes evident during exercise lasting longer than one to two hours, especially in the heat. The carbohydrates contained in sports drinks help reduce the utilization of muscle glycogen, which can help improve exercise performance. It is important to note that not all sport drinks are alike. Some, in fact, may just be glorified sugar water. When choosing sports drinks, look for those containing less than 8% carbohydrate.[30] Beverages containing high doses of simple sugars may slow the absorption of the fluid, which may decrease exercise performance. The type of carbohydrate used in sports drinks may also be a factor to consider. For example, high levels of fructose in drinks may promote slower absorption than drinks containing other sugars such as glucose.

Glutamine

Glutamine is an amino acid—one of the building blocks that make up protein. Glutamine is usually labeled a *non-essential* amino acid, because we have the ability to make it as needed. However, it appears that our need for glutamine may increase under certain conditions such as surgery or chronic, debilitating disease. It is for this reason that glutamine is sometimes called a *conditionally essential amino acid*. Research finds that when glutamine is given intravenously to sick people, it may help improve body weight and muscle mass and reduce the time one spends in the hospital.[74] Some wonder whether this effect might also be experienced by healthy people who exercise, but research has not observed that glutamine improves strength or athletic performance in healthy populations.[75]

Many athletes such as bodybuilders use glutamine not to make them stronger, but rather to slow muscle breakdown and speed up the time required to recover following repeated bouts of high-intensity exercise. Though this might be possible, sound scientific evidence to support this theory is lacking. Some research has noted that orally ingested glutamine, when used in conjunction with the amino acid arginine and a supplement called HMB, may hold promise for reducing muscle loss in those with cancer and HIV.[76] Whether or not similar results would be experienced by healthy people such as bodybuilders remains unknown. For additional information, see my blog post "Glutamine: The Dirty Little Secret" at Supplement-Geek.com.

Blood Doping

Blood doping, which involves donating and storing one's own blood, is a dangerous practice used by some elite cyclists and marathoners. After being stored for a period of time, the blood is then pumped back into the athlete's body before a race or event in order to boost the concentration of oxygen-carrying red blood cells. More red blood cells yield a greater oxygen-carrying capacity, which in turn may foster one's ability to exercise longer and at a higher intensity. One of the problems with blood doping is that when athletes exercise, they tend to sweat. This loss of fluid from the body means the blood gets thicker, which places added stress on the heart as it works harder to pump the thicker blood. Heart attacks and death have been known to occur following blood doping, and for this reason, it is illegal in many sports.

Another strategy sometimes employed is to use a drug called EPO, a synthetic version of erythropoietin, which is a hormone that makes red blood cells. When an individual uses EPO, red blood cell production increases, resulting in increased blood viscosity, a condition that can be hazardous to health for the same reasons mentioned previously. The use of EPO is also illegal in most sports.

Training at Higher Altitudes

When preparing for a race or other athletic event, some athletes train in places situated at higher altitudes than the event's location. At higher altitudes, less oxygen is generally available for the person to breathe. Consequently, the body must adapt to the lack of oxygen by naturally making more red blood cells (erythrocytes). When the athlete returns to lower elevations, he or she may have more stamina and improved exercise performance because of their greater oxygen carrying capacity. Keep in mind that increases in red blood cell levels do not occur overnight. Rather, several weeks of living and exercising at higher altitudes may be needed before significant changes are observed.

Another consideration when training at higher altitudes involves the increased use of protein for fuel that might occur as a result of the body burning more calories than it normally does at lower elevations, which could result in muscle loss and reduced exercise performance. Increased calorie needs may also be expected if the athlete trains at a higher altitude featuring temperatures that are colder than normal. These caveats notwithstanding, training at higher altitudes has been called *natural blood doping* by some because of its ability to boost performance. Training at higher altitudes, however, unlike authentic blood doping, is not an illegal practice.

Vitamin B$_{12}$ Supplements

Vitamin B$_{12}$ is needed for the production of red blood cells, which carry oxygen. Thus, like other practices described above, the rationale behind using vitamin B$_{12}$ supplements is that the nutrient might boost red blood cell production, which, in turn, has the potential to improve exercise performance. However, research has not yet demonstrated that exercise ability improves following vitamin B$_{12}$ supplementation in healthy people. It is noteworthy to mention that, unlike many of the regularly excreted B vitamins, vitamin B_{12} is stored for a few years in the body. Thus, deficiencies in this vitamin are unlikely, especially in athletes and regular exercisers who are not vegetarians, who eat a healthy diet, or who use supplements containing this nutrient.

Iron Supplements

The mineral iron is crucial for red blood cells to carry oxygen. As such, some people may use iron supplements in the hopes that it will help their blood transport more oxygen, battle exercise fatigue, and improve overall exercise capacity. For those who have been diagnosed with iron-deficiency anemia, iron supplements may, in fact, be helpful for improving overall health and exercise performance. For those who are not anemic, however, iron supplements do not appear offer significant benefits. When used in excess, iron can actually be dangerous, especially for those with a rare genetic condition called *hemochromotosis* (iron overload disease). In this disorder, iron absorption is enhanced, leading to a wide spectrum of problems ranging from joint pain and fatigue to liver disorders and even death. Iron is also a controversial mineral for men, as some research suggests that excess iron could be a possible contributor to heart disease. For this reason, many men's formula multi-vitamins do not contain iron. Iron is found in meats as well as many green vegetables and legumes. Unless prescribed by a doctor, iron supplements cannot be recommended.

Sodium Bicarbonate

The letters pH refer to a 0–14 scale that is often used in chemistry to measure acidity levels. Lower pH numbers indicate greater acidity, while higher numbers reflect alkalinity. Metabolic acids produced during exercise can decrease exercise performance by inducing fatigue and reducing muscular power capacity. Given this fact, some athletes may attempt to protect the body against increases in acid production for the purpose of extending the time before fatigue sets in. Normally this practice involves the use of baking soda (sodium bicarbonate) before an athletic event. Research, while mixed, does hint that sodium bicarbonate may be of help to athletes involved not only in highly anaerobic types of activity such as sprinting, but also to those who participate in marathons and triathlons. Bicarbonate is typically used 1–2 hours before a competition at a concentration of about 300 milligrams per kilogram of body weight.[79] Some research suggests that this practice may help shave a few seconds off of an athlete's time, which in competitive events, is significant. An individual considering sodium bicarbonate should experiment with it before the actual athletic event to see how his or her body responds. Studies indicate that sodium bicarbonate may cause diarrhea and abdominal pain 1–2 hours after ingestion.

For more info on other exercise products, see my website, www.Supplement-Geek.com.

Chapter 6

Vitamins & Minerals

Vitamins

Vitamins are organic compounds needed in small amounts to ensure health. The term *organic* refers to the fact that vitamins contain the element carbon, which is fundamental to all life on earth. To be classified as a vitamin, the substance in question must either:

1. not be naturally made in the body

2. be associated with a disease or condition when missing from the diet

The classic example often used to illustrate these characteristics of vitamins is the story of vitamin C. Hundreds of years ago, British sailors on long sea voyages frequently developed scurvy, a condition that, if not corrected, is fatal. In time, it was discovered that eating citrus fruits prevented scurvy. Thus, limes and other citrus fruits came into widespread use by sailors in the British Navy. Ultimately, the compound in citrus fruits that prevented scurvy was discovered to be vitamin C. Interestingly, British sailors earned the popular nickname "limeys" because of their dependence on limes for this crucial vitamin.

As mentioned above, the body generally cannot make vitamins. Thus, vitamins must either be obtained from food or through the use of supplements. The exception to this rule is vitamin D, which can be made upon exposure to sunlight. Vitamins can be classified according to whether they dissolve in fat or water. While fat-soluble vitamins include vitamins A, E, D, and K, the water-soluble vitamins are vitamin C and the B complex family of vitamins.

The Fat-Soluble Vitamins

Vitamins A, E, D, and K are fat-soluble vitamins. They are called fat-soluble because they are best absorbed when consumed with some fat. This is one of the reasons why it is sometimes recommended that multivitamins be taken with meals.

The fat-soluble vitamins serve an array of purposes. For example, vitamin A aids with the proper functioning of the eyes.[36] Vitamin E helps blood circulate more freely throughout the body by reducing the likelihood of blood clots. Vitamin K, on the other hand, helps blood to clot in the event of a cut or injury. Lastly, one function of vitamin D is that it helps with proper bone development.

Because the human body is able to store fat-soluble vitamins for great lengths of time (years in some cases), they do not need to be ingested daily.[36] In fact, due to the possibility of toxic reactions, medical professionals typically discourage patients from ingesting fat-soluble vitamins in excess of their recommended dietary allowance. For example, pregnant women who consume large amounts of vitamin A early in their pregnancy increase the chances that their infant may have birth defects.[36] In children, high intakes of vitamin A can result in itchy skin, swelling of the bones, and irritability.[36] In adults, high vitamin A consumption can result in nausea, drowsiness, hair loss, diarrhea, and the loss of calcium from the bones.[36] Fortunately, a reversal of these symptoms occurs once vitamin A consumption returns to recommended levels.[36] With regard to vitamin D, kidney damage and weaker bones have been linked with high intakes of this vitamin.[36] Vitamin K ingested in excess has the potential to affect the blood's clotting ability and may negatively interact with blood thinner medications. Some research, albeit controversial, has even noted higher rates of death associated with vitamin E in excess of 400 IUs per day.[77]

Vitamin A

Vitamin A was given its name because it was the very first fat-soluble vitamin discovered. While mostly known to help prevent night blindness, vitamin A is also important for maintaining the immune system and for supporting proper bone development. As mentioned previously, high levels of vitamin A can become toxic, resulting in a number of side effects, the most serious of which is liver damage. Birth defects are also possible if high levels of vitamin A are ingested during pregnancy. Furthermore, vitamin A supplements may increase osteoporosis risk in postmenopausal women.[136] Some research even finds that high-dose vitamin A supplements may increase death rate.[135] To avert these hazards, multivitamin supplements usually contain beta-carotene in place of vitamin A. The body can make vitamin A from beta-carotene but does so in a way that avoids its buildup to toxic levels. Because of the risks associated with overconsumption, one should always consult a physician before using vitamin A supplements.

What Is Beta-Carotene?

Beta-carotene is a member of the carotenoid family of phytonutrients and is found in foods such as carrots and sweet potatoes. Many multivitamins contain beta-carotene instead of vitamin A because too much vitamin A can damage the liver. The body can convert beta-carotene into vitamin A and does so in a way that prevents vitamin A from building up to toxic levels. Some people may also use beta-carotene supplements because they believe that it has anti-cancer or anti-heart disease properties. The rationale for this is that beta-carotene is found in fruits and vegetables, and people who eat these foods regularly tend to be less likely to develop heart disease, cancer, ,and a host of other illnesses. However, when beta-carotene was tested to see if it could protect people from disease, it not only failed, but was found to promote lung cancer in smokers and in those who worked around asbestos.[80] Because several studies have come to the same conclusion, it is generally recommend that smokers and asbestos-exposed workers avoid beta-carotene supplements. How beta-carotene promotes lung cancer is not well-understood. It is worth mentioning that eating foods that contain beta-carotene has never been shown to promote lung cancer or any other harmful condition. Foods contain hundreds of carotenoids, beta-carotene, and other compounds that probably work together when eaten. The case of beta-carotene is something fitness professionals would be wise to remember when discussing high doses of individual nutrients with clients.

Vitamin E

Since its discovery almost one hundred years ago, fat-soluble vitamin E (alpha tocopherol) has not only been one of the most popular vitamins, but has also been one of the most controversial. The term *vitamin E* actually refers to a family of eight related compounds. They are alpha, beta, gamma and delta tocopherol and alpha, beta, gamma and delta tocotrienol. Alpha tocopherol is the type most often found in multivitamins and is the most abundant type in the human body.

Most interest in vitamin E revolves around its antioxidant capabilities. Antioxidants are molecules that neutralize free radicals, which are normally-produced atoms and molecules which, in excess, are thought to disrupt normal cell operations and contribute to disease. This has lead to the widespread use of vitamin E supplements in an attempt to ward off free radical production and to reduce the risk of various conditions such as heart disease.

Despite its popularity, vitamin E remains controversial due to conflicting evidence substantiating its impact on heart disease and other ailments. While some evidence suggests synthetic vitamin E may slow the progression of Alzheimer's disease, the vitamin does not appear to stop Alzheimer's from occurring.[137,138] Conversely, other recent data suggests that increased death rates may be associated with high intakes of this vitamin.[80] Because vitamin E has "blood thinning" properties, it could potentially interact with blood thinner medications and should therefore be avoided unless prescribed by a physician.

Vitamin D

Vitamin D is a nutrient that is based on cholesterol and is made when the body is exposed to sunlight. This vitamin is also found in fortified dairy products such as milk and yogurt. Vitamin D is most often mentioned in conjunction with calcium, because it helps the body absorb this mineral. As such, vitamin D can help keep bones strong and offset osteoporosis. Emerging research, though, suggests that vitamin D may have other uses as well. For example, several studies have found that vitamin D may reduce the incidence of falls in older adults by over 20%.[84] Other research suggests that reduced vitamin D may increase the risk of some cancers, multiple sclerosis, and rheumatoid arthritis.[139]

Supplements usually contain either vitamin D2 (ergocalciferol), which is plant-based, or vitamin D$_3$ (cholecalciferol), which is similar to what the body generates from sunlight and is thought to be more potent. Our ability to make vitamin D from sunlight tends to decline as we get older. This, along with the fact that many seniors may not get outside as much as they did when they were younger, could accelerate osteoporosis. Likewise, obese individuals may also be vitamin D-deficient.[140]

One cup of milk contains about 100 IU of vitamin D. The nutrient is also found in some calcium supplements to enhance calcium absorption. The RDA for vitamin D is 600 IU. When discussing the health benefits of vitamin D, fitness professionals should keep in mind that vitamin D can interact negatively with various diseases and medications that people may be taking. When in doubt, refer to a registered dietitian, doctor, or pharmacist, who can discuss supplement-drug interactions and their possible impact of a variety of diseases and conditions.

Vitamin K

Like vitamin D, the body has a way of obtaining vitamin K internally, thanks to the help of bacteria living in the human digestive track. Vitamin K is one of the many players in the complex cascade of events that allow the blood to in case of injury. Without vitamin K, a simple cut on a finger could be life-threatening! Aside from this crucial role, other research hints that vitamin K may also be needed to maintain bone strength. Vitamin K supplements are usually not needed by healthy people because it is produced by intestinal bacteria. This vitamin is also readily available in green leafy vegetables. Because of its ability to help blood clot, one side effect often associated with vitamin K is its possible interaction with blood thinner medications.

Fat Soluble Vitamins

Vitamin	Selected Function	Sources	Signs of Excess
Vitamin A	Vision	Sweet potatoes, carrots, spinach	Fatigue, irritability, abdominal pain
Vitamin E	Antioxidant	Green leafy vegetables, nuts	Nausea, fatigue
Vitamin D	Calcium absorption	Sunlight, fortified dairy products	Weaker bones, fatigue
Vitamin K	Blood clotting	Intestinal bacteria, soy, green leafy vegetables	Blood clots

The Water-Soluble Vitamins

The water-soluble vitamins include vitamins C and the B-complex family of vitamins. The B vitamins can sometimes be difficult to remember because some are referred to by their B vitamin number while others are called by alternate names. For example, vitamin B_{12} is often identified by letter and number, while others tend to be referred to by their more popular names. The B-complex family of vitamins include vitamin B_1 (thiamine), vitamin B_2 (riboflavin), vitamin B_3 (niacin), vitamin B_5 (pantothenic acid), vitamin B_6 (pyridoxine), vitamin B_{12} (cyanocobalamin), vitamin B_9 (folate, folacin, or folic acid), and biotin. Inositol (sometimes called "vitamin B_8") is sometimes grouped among the B vitamins, but it is made in the body and is usually not regarded as an essential nutrient.

Unlike the fat-soluble vitamins, water-soluble vitamins are not stored in the body for great lengths of time.[36] Unless they are supplied by food or vitamin supplements, deficiencies in many water-soluble vitamins can become evident after only 4 weeks.[36]

For the most part, the water-soluble vitamins work with enzymes, which are biological machines or *catalysts* that accelerate chemical reactions in the body. Were it not for digestive enzymes, it might take years for the body to fully digest your last meal.

Energy-generating reactions are central to many of the functions of the B vitamins. For example, in the event that insufficient carbohydrates are available, the body can transform protein into glucose to help meet its energy needs. This process is called *gluconeogenesis* and requires vitamin B_6. In addition, B vitamins are needed not only for the storage of fat and glycogen, but also for their aerobic and anaerobic breakdown. In spite of their function in energy-generating pathways, vitamins do not provide energy directly. The simple reason for this is that vitamins contain no usable calories (energy). Thus, adding B vitamins to energy drinks serves little purpose and does not provide an authentic "energy boost" for most people.

With respect to exercise, studies generally find that consuming excess water-soluble vitamins (or any vitamins for that matter) does not improve exercise performance in healthy, well-nourished individuals. This is the reason why most nutrition experts refrain from recommending much more than a multivitamin to athletes and exercisers who already eat a healthy diet.

Thiamin

Thiamin is the more recognizable name for vitamin B_1. One of the classic thiamin-deficiency syndromes is called *beriberi*—a disease that can lead to paralysis, nerve damage, and death. However, thiamin deficiency in the US is rare because flour and grains are usually fortified with this vitamin during processing. Because it is usually consumed in normal, healthy diets, thiamin supplements are usually not needed.

Some people who exercise may supplement with thiamin. The rationale for this is that a thiamin deficiency could lead to elevations in lactate, which is correlated with muscle burning and reductions in the amount of force that muscles can generate during exercise. Thus, lactate accumulation has the potential to reduce exercise performance. Whether or not supplemental thiamin can improve exercise performance in those who are not thiamin deficient is not well studied. Good sources of thiamin include lean pork, enriched breads, and many fortified breakfast cereals.

Riboflavin

Riboflavin, also called vitamin B_2, was first found in milk in the late 1870s. While required for proper energy production, riboflavin is also needed to help other vitamins such as folic acid, niacin, and B_6 to work properly. Emerging research also hints that riboflavin may help reduce the incidence of migraine headaches.[85]

Riboflavin is a rather delicate vitamin and is easily destroyed by sunlight. This is the reason why many milk containers are not clear plastic. The name "riboflavin" stems from its yellow color. In fact, high intakes of riboflavin are one reason why most urine appears at least slightly yellow. Riboflavin is usually found in dairy products and green vegetables. Many cereal and grain products are also fortified with this nutrient.

Niacin

Niacin is also called vitamin B$_3$. Another name that refers to niacin is *nicotinic acid*. The classic deficiency condition associated with niacin is *pellagra*, which results in scaly, dry skin as well as damage to the central nervous system. Pellagra was common in the early 20th century but is relatively uncommon in the US today because many foods are fortified with this vitamin. The body also has the ability to make niacin from the amino acid tryptophan. Because of their poor dietary habits, however, alcoholics are one group in which pellagra may still occur.

Niacin normally helps the body carry out many crucial functions required for optimal health, including the production of glycogen and the breakdown of fat for fuel. High levels of niacin (more than the RDA) might also reduce cholesterol and triglycerides and have the ability to boost good cholesterol (HDL) concentrations. Physicians may prescribe high-dose niacin for this reason. Ongoing research also hints that high doses of niacin may hold promise for staving off cataracts, diabetes, and heart disease.[87, 88, 89]

People with high cholesterol may gravitate toward taking niacin supplements because they want to try a natural treatment before opting to use medications. These individuals must remember that high doses of niacin are not without risks. For example, some research finds that high intakes of niacin (1–3 g per day) may increase homocysteine by as much as 55%.[86] Homocysteine is thought to be a contributor to heart disease risk. Other research finds that niacin can also damage the liver in some cases.

Some evidence suggests that vitamin C, vitamin E, and beta-carotene appear to block niacin's ability to elevate HDL.[90] This may hinder those with cholesterol problems from getting the most out of niacin therapy. High-dose niacin may also be inappropriate for those with diabetes because of its potential to elevate blood sugar levels. While definitely needed in small amounts to maintain optimal health, high-dose niacin supplements should only be used by those under the care of a physician. For healthy persons, there is not enough evidence to recommend niacin supplements. Good sources of niacin include meats and beans as well as foods fortified with this nutrient.

Pantothenic Acid

Pantothenic acid, also known as vitamin B$_5$, helps the body burn fats and carbohydrates and extracts energy from protein when necessary. Pantothenic acid is also needed for the production of acetylcholine, a neurotransmitter needed for all muscle contraction. It is because of the vitamin's production of acetylcholine that some exercisers may supplement with pantothenic acid. Research to date, while limited, has not observed any significant effect of this vitamin on exercise ability. Like other B vitamins, pantothenic acid is found in many fortified foods, so deficiency is rare in healthy people eating a well-balanced diet.

Foods rich in pantothenic acid include poultry and other meats, legumes, and whole grains. Pantothenic acid is also found in some shampoos. This may be due to the belief by some that the vitamin could prevent hair from turning gray or falling out, though this claim appears baseless.

People considering pantothenic acid supplements should take note that only the "right-handed" or "d" version can be used by the body. Thus, supplements may list the vitamin as "d-pantothenic acid".

Vitamin B_6

Vitamin B_6, also called *pyridoxine*, takes part in over one hundred biochemical reactions required for the body to function. For example, the body has the ability to make non-essential amino acids like glutamine and arginine because of vitamin B_6. In fact, Vitamin B_6 is needed to make all of the non-essential amino acids. This vitamin is also required to transform amino acids into glucose through the process called "gluconeogenesis." Of all the uses of this vitamin, the one that seems to garner most attention is its ability to lower homocysteine, an amino acid linked to the development of heart disease. The vitamins folic acid and vitamin B_{12} also lower homocysteine levels and may appear together in supplements specifically marketed to those interested in heart health. Keep in mind that this is controversial and lowering homocysteine may not necessarily reduce the risk of heart disease.

Another marker of heart disease is an inflammation-related molecule called "C reactive protein" (CRP). CRP levels tend to rise in response to infections, and research is being gathered to demonstrate that chronically elevated CRP may damage blood vessels in a way that makes them susceptible to the development of artery-clogging plaque. Some research finds that low pyridoxine levels may also contribute to higher CRP concentrations.[91]

Vitamin B_6 is generally considered safe when consumed in quantities lower than the RDA. High doses over long periods of time might cause nerve damage and, as such, should only be used under the supervision of a physician. Good sources of vitamin B_6 include bananas, fish, eggs, poultry, and meats.

Folate

Folate, a term derived from a Latin word that means "leaf" (as in leafy vegetables), is also known as "folacin" and "vitamin B_9." *Folic acid* is the synthetic form of folate. All terms are usually used interchangeably. Folic acid is needed for the production of DNA, our "genetic blueprint" or "software program." For this reason, folic acid is incorporated to prenatal vitamins to helps prevent birth defects. Folic acid is also needed to make the hemoglobin portion of oxygen-carrying red blood cells. Thus, deficiencies in folic acid could result in anemia. Furthermore, folic acid lowers homocysteine.

This vitamin is often added to breakfast cereals and is also found naturally in leafy green vegetables, such as broccoli and spinach, as well as bananas. One group in whom folic acid supplements might be inappropriate includes those with epilepsy and other seizure disorders. Some research hints that, in these individuals, folic acid supplements might enhance seizure rate.[82] The synthetic version of this vitamin (folic acid) is more bioavailable than folate (the natural form). Therefore, most multivitamins contain folic acid rather than folate.

Vitamin B_{12}

Other names for vitamin B_{12} are "cyanocobalamin" and "methylcobalamin." Unlike other B vitamins that are found in various amounts in meats and vegetables, vitamin B_{12} is only found in meats.

Some older adults may go to their physician to receive injections of vitamin B_{12}, particularly because elderly populations may sometimes have difficulty absorbing this nutrient. *Intrinsic factor* is a molecule produced by the stomach that helps us absorb vitamin B_{12}. In addition to advancing age, undergoing stomach or intestinal surgery might also reduce intrinsic factor production, which in turn limits vitamin B_{12} absorption. Reduced stomach acid production, which may arise in people who take antacids on a regular basis, might also reduce B_{12} absorption. Injections of B_{12} can bypass this problem. Vitamin B_{12} can also be absorbed from the small intestine, although this rout is less efficient.

The liver can actually store vitamin B_{12} for several years. In some cases, the body can be so efficient at storing vitamin B_{12} that deficiency symptoms may not become evident for 5 years![93] Signs of vitamin B_{12} deficiency include anemia, fatigue, dementia, and, if not corrected, irreversible brain damage.[92]

Vitamin B_{12} may be used by people who exercise because some believe that it enhances energy. Athletes may even get injections of this vitamin in the hopes of supercharging their systems and boosting red blood cell production. Research thus far, however, has not found that vitamin B_{12} supplements can enhance exercise performance in those who are not deficient in this nutrient.

With respect to overall health, vitamin B_{12} can reduce homocysteine, which, as described previously, may influence the risk of heart disease. Folic acid and vitamin B_6 also reduce homocysteine levels. Aside from seniors, strict vegetarians or vegans are also at risk for vitamin B_{12} deficiency. While vegetarians and vegans can obtain adequate protein by combining different plant-based foods, it is often difficult for them to ingest sufficient amounts of vitamin B_{12} without using a vitamin supplement.

Biotin

Biotin is occasionally called "vitamin H," but it is a water-soluble vitamin and is generally listed as a member of the B-complex family. Biotin helps the body use fats, carbohydrates, and proteins and also helps the immune system function. This vitamin is stored in the mitochondria, the cellular site of fat-burning and, when eaten, has a very high absorption rate. Biotin is found naturally in cauliflower, peanut butter, and soybeans. Additionally, bacteria inside the body make this nutrient. Thus, biotin deficiency is highly unlikely.

Biotin is sometimes found in hair products, probably because of the belief that it can prevent hair from falling out. Though hair loss is a symptom of biotin deficiency, research to date has not revealed that adding extra biotin prevents hair loss in healthy people.

Vitamin C

Like many of the B vitamins, vitamin C, the other water-soluble vitamin, is not stored in great amounts in the body. Vitamin C (ascorbic acid) is an antioxidant and therefore helps protect against cellular damage caused by free radicals. It is also indispensable to the proper formation of connective tissue.

Vitamin C may be used by some to prevent colds, although research to date has not shown that it truly has this ability. Studies do find, however, that if taken at the first sign of a cold, vitamin C may reduce (by a couple days) the duration of cold symptoms. This is one of the most controversial aspects of vitamin C research, as not all research supports this finding.[94]

Regardless of its effects on the common cold, vitamin C does appear to exert influences beyond its previously mentioned ability to prevent and cure scurvy. Vitamin C is needed for the production of cartilage and may help slow the rate of destruction of cartilage.[96] Because the wearing way of cartilage has the potential to cause osteoarthritis, vitamin C may help prevent the development of this condition. Research also suggests that vitamin C may reduce the risk of some types of cancer, including those of the mouth and stomach.[94] Furthermore, vitamin C may help keep bones strong.[96]

In athletes such as long distance runners and triathletes, a well-documented suppression of the immune system may occur as a result of heavy training schedules and stress to the body during the event, which can leave the athlete prone to infections in the days following the race. Some research finds vitamin C taken several days prior to a race may bolster the immune system enough to reduce this risk.[97]

With respect to side effects, vitamin C is known to increase the absorption of iron, and too much absorbed iron may contribute to diseases such as diabetes, heart and liver disease, and some types of cancer.[36] In people with a genetic condition called *iron overload disease* (also called "hemochromotosis"), too much iron is already absorbed. In these individuals, vitamin C supplements may make their condition worse. DRelated to this, some research suggests that men with high levels of iron in their blood may be at increased risk of heart disease.[48] For this reason, some men's formula multivitamins do not contain iron.

For those desiring to experiment with vitamin C, keep in mind that the body absorbs this nutrient most efficiently at low doses. The higher the dose in a supplement, the less vitamin C the body absorbs.

Antioxidants like vitamin C are very popular among people desiring to reduce their risk of cancer. While the evidence for this is far from resolved, the use of antioxidant supplements by people undergoing cancer treatments such as chemotherapy should be discussed with an oncologist. While more research is needed, some speculate that antioxidants might decrease the effectiveness of chemo therapy.[98]

The Water Soluble Vitamins

Vitamin	Selected Functions	Good Sources	Signs of Excess
Vitamin C	Antioxidant; aids with proper formation of connective tissue	Citrus fruits, broccoli, green peppers, strawberries	Kidney stones, iron overload disease
Vitamin B_1/Thiamin	Aids with carbohydrate breakdown	Yeast, pork, beans	Dermatitis
Vitamin B_2/Riboflavin	Participates in aerobic metabolism	Beef liver, steak, cheese	Yellow/orange discoloration of urine
Vitamin B_6	Helps with protein synthesis and glycogen metabolism; helps with hemoglobin synthesis	Brewers yeast, lima beans, beef liver	Nausea, vomiting, reversible nerve damage
Vitamin B_{12}	Helps with protein synthesis; helps lower homocysteine; helps with proper red blood cell formation	Meat, fish, milk, poultry	Diarrhea
Niacin	Helps with aerobic and anaerobic metabolism; helps with both fat and glycogen synthesis	Tuna, beef, chicken	Headache, nausea, vomiting, diarrhea, blurred vision, liver toxicity
Pantothenic acid	Helps with aerobic metabolism; helps with synthesis of red blood cells	Egg yoke, yeast, intestinal bacteria	Diarrhea

Folic Acid	Helps with red blood cell formation; lowers homocysteine; lowers neural tube defects	Steak, bananas, salmon	Irritability, excitability, confusion
Biotin	Helps with fat synthesis	Yeast, egg yoke, liver, kidney	None reported

Vitamins and Exercise Performance

Multivitamin supplements are the most common form of supplements used by Americans, representing between 70–90% of all products purchased.[36] There is no doubt that the human body requires a wide array of vitamins to function properly. For example, vitamin B_{12} is needed for the proper formation of red blood cells; vitamin C is required for the development of connective tissue (collagen); and vitamin D helps calcium absorption. Given their crucial role in health, one might wonder whether vitamins enhance exercise performance. Unfortunately, this does not seem to be the case. Research since the 1950s has not shown that vitamin supplements improve exercise performance in healthy, well nourished men or women.[36] In fact, a review of over 90 scientific studies concluded that the vitamin needs of both athletes and non-athletes are rather similar.[17] Some vitamins do take part in chemical reactions involved in energy metabolism. This may have spawned the idea that vitamin supplements provide energy or "pep" during exercise, which is generally untrue. Vitamins do not provide any energy directly because they have no usable calories. Studies of exercising individuals have shown that as physical activity increases, so also does the amount of food (and thus, calories and nutrients) that is consumed.[36] Thus, physically active people already tend to be better nourished than non-exercising individuals. For those who wish to have the added "insurance" of a multivitamin, remember that, as a general rule, cheaper multivitamins are probably just as effective as more expensive brands.

Natural vs. Synthetic Vitamins

Studies have repeatedly shown that synthetic vitamins made in the laboratory are of the same quality as those made in nature. This makes sense, because the molecular structures of both synthetic and natural vitamins are identical, so the body cannot tell the difference between them.

The case for vitamin E is one classic example often used in an attempt to prove the superiority of natural over synthetic vitamins. It turns out that the body does utilize natural vitamin E better than synthetic vitamin E—and for a very good reason. Just as some people in the world are left-handed and others are right-handed, the same is also true for molecules! Technically, we refer to left-handed molecules as *levorotatory* (or "L" for short). Right-handed molecules are given the name *dextrorotatory* (or "D" for short). The human body prefers right-handed (D) vitamin E over left-hand (L) vitamin E. Thus, theoretically, natural vitamin E would be composed of all right-handed molecules (i.e., only the d version). Synthetic vitamin E is actually composed of a mixture of both right- and left-handed molecules (referred to as "dl alpha tocopherol" on many multivitamin labels), of which we can only use the right-handed version. So, in theory, only 50% of synthetic vitamin E can be utilized by the body. It should be noted, however, that right-handed vitamin E made in the laboratory is absorbed no differently than right-handed vitamin E made in nature's laboratory.

Vitamins as Antioxidants

Many vitamins function in the body as *antioxidants*. Antioxidants are compounds that neutralize highly reactive, damaging atoms and molecules called *free radicals*. Free radicals combine with other molecules and atoms and, in the process, disrupt normal cellular operation. Free radicals are thought to cause and contribute to a variety of diseases and conditions ranging from heart disease and cancer to the very aging process itself. The vitamins, A, C, and vitamin E are classic examples of vitamins that function as antioxidants. It should be mentioned that the beneficial effects attributed to single antioxidants might be the result of the interaction between several different molecules in food. For example, some studies show an increased risk of lung cancer when smokers take beta-carotene supplements.[59] These findings hint that the beneficial effect attributed to beta-carotene may, in fact, be the result of its interaction with other nutrients in food. This, along with other facts, supports the notion that people should obtain antioxidants from food whenever possible. Given that we may have not have yet discovered all of the nutrients in a given food, this is sage advice. If unknown components of food do exist, they may inadvertently be left out of the processing of supplements. Currently, research is also being done to uncover the effects of various plant chemicals (phytonutrients) and the role they play in disease prevention.

The Minerals

The minerals are a group of inorganic compounds that, like vitamins, are required for the maintenance of health. Minerals are called inorganic because they do not contain the element carbon. They help with a variety of functions needed for optimal health. For example, iron is needed by every red blood cell in the body and is crucial for the production of hemoglobin, the oxygen-carrying component of red blood cells. Calcium, while normally only considered when talking about bone strength, is crucial to all muscle contraction as well as blood clotting. The mineral phosphorous is a part of every ATP molecule, and magnesium is needed to extract the energy from ATP. Moreover, no life on earth would be possible if it were not for sodium and potassium, which together are fundamental to both the conduction of nerve impulses as well as all muscle contractions.

The minerals can be subdivided into two groups: the *major minerals*—which are required in amounts of more than 100 mg—and the *trace* minerals, which are needed in amounts of less than 100 mg.[36]

Boron

The trace mineral boron used to be utilized as a food preservative. Today boron is mostly used as a supplement or is found in supplements along with other ingredients. Boron is sometimes touted to help a number of conditions, but more research is needed to verify most claims. For example, some research suggests that boron may help keep bones strong, but the evidence is not as definitive as for that of calcium. Strength trainers used to take boron supplements because it was believed that the mineral could boost testosterone levels. Research does show that boron may help raise testosterone—if you are an older women who has been put on a boron-deficient diet. Research conducted on healthy men and women who strength train, however, has not noted significant elevations in testosterone or strength following boron supplementation. Boron is found naturally in green leafy vegetables, apples, nuts, and beans.

Calcium

When most people think of calcium, they almost automatically think of bones—and for good reason. Upwards of 99% of the body's calcium is contained in the bones and teeth, where it provides strength, a term technically referred to as *bone mineral density* (BMD). Aside from helping keep bones strong, calcium has other uses as well. For example, calcium is involved in muscle contraction, nerve impulse transmission, and blood clotting. There are even calcium-containing adhesive molecules called *cadherins* that act like glue and help our cells to stick together.

Another issue where calcium may play a role is weight loss. Some intriguing research has hinted that calcium-rich dairy products, in association with a reduced calorie diet, may help reduce weight.[100] To determine whether or not calcium supplements produce the same results, more study is needed.

Because most of the body's calcium resides in the bones and teeth, these places serve as reservoirs from which the body can draw calcium during times when it does not get adequate levels of this mineral from the diet. The problem with this is that, as the body removes calcium from these areas, they become weaker. Supplemental calcium may be something to consider because research finds that some Americans may not ingest enough of this mineral.

When choosing a calcium supplement, it is important to consider *elemental calcium*, which is the calcium that we use. Different types of calcium contain different amounts of elemental calcium. Thus, a 500 mg calcium supplement may not contain 500 mg of elemental calcium. The amount of elemental calcium contained in a supplement may or may not be listed on the product's label. Of all calcium types, *calcium carbonate* has the most elemental calcium (40%). *Calcium citrate* has the next highest (21%). *Calcium lactate* has about 13% elemental calcium and *calcium gluconate* has about 9% elemental calcium. Determining how much elemental calcium contained in a supplement is just a matter of multiplying the milligrams of calcium in the supplement by its corresponding percent of elemental calcium. For example, a 500 mg calcium carbonate supplement can be expected to have 500mg X .40 = 200 mg of elemental calcium. A 500 mg calcium citrate supplement has 500 x .21 = 105 mg of elemental calcium.

As mentioned previously, long-term lack of dietary calcium can result in *osteoporosis*. Osteoporosis affects more than 25 million Americans, with the majority being older women.[38] Osteoporosis arises when bone is lost faster than it is made. While traditionally thought of as a condition that only affects older people, osteoporosis is increasingly being viewed as a disease that starts when we are young. This is highlighted by the fact that bone loss begins around the age of 35.[11] The National Institute of Health (NIH) has recommended that adolescent girls consume 1500 mg of calcium per day.[36] In addition, osteoporosis affects men, in whom it contributes to an estimated 10,000 hip fractures each year.[38] Risk factors for osteoporosis include:

1. **Race**. Caucasians and those of Asian decent are at greater risk.
2. **Gender**. Women have a 4 times greater risk of osteoporosis.
3. **Family history**. Risk increases if family members also have osteoporosis.
4. **Age**. Osteoporosis increases as we age.
5. **Early menopause**. Risk increases in those who experience menopause earlier than expected.
6. **Lifestyle behaviors**. Smoking, alcohol abuse, lack of dietary calcium, high intakes of caffeine or salt, lack of exercise, and drinking more than 2 cups of coffee per day all appear to increase risk.

Fiber is one of the nutrients known to inhibit calcium absorption. Thus, people on high-fiber diets may want to separate fiber-containing meals from calcium supplements by a few hours to enhance absorption. Natural sources of calcium include not only milk and other dairy products, but also soy, broccoli, boney fish, and some mineral waters. Calcium may be added to some commercial orange juices as well.

Chromium

The essential trace mineral chromium is most well known because of its effect on blood sugar. Chromium helps insulin work better and, as such, may be of help to some pre-diabetics by helping stabilize blood sugar. Chromium is sometimes called *glucose tolerance factor* (GTF) because of its blood sugar-lowering effect, although technically this is not true—chromium is part of the GTF molecule but by itself is not GTF. Chromium is often found in weight loss supplements, but most research to date does not show that it helps.[60] Natural sources of chromium include meats, brewer's yeast, rye bread, fish, and tea. For more on chromium see the chapter on dietary supplements.

Copper

The essential trace mineral copper is needed to make oxygen-carrying red blood cells and to help several enzymes function properly. For example, copper is required to make a mitochondrial enzyme called cytochrome-c oxidase, which is crucial for ATP production. That being said, copper deficiency is rare and supplements are generally not needed. Copper supplements could be dangerous and could damage the liver. Additionally, the mineral zinc can interfere with copper absorption. This may be something to consider if using zinc to battle colds. Natural sources of copper include meats, nuts, legumes, and seafood.

Iodine

The mineral iodine is essential for metabolism. One of the key players in metabolic rate is thyroid hormone. For thyroid hormone to function, it must have iodine. In fact, iodine is so crucial that most of this mineral is stored in the thyroid gland! One classic sign of an iodine deficiency is an enlargement of the thyroid gland, a condition referred to as a *goiter*. Iodine deficiency in the US is unlikely, however. Much of the table salt used in US households today is iodized to prevent iodine deficiency. Some weight loss supplements may also contain iodine, presumably in the hopes of boosting metabolism via increasing thyroid hormone. This may not work however if the person is not deficient in iodine. Besides table salt, good sources of iodine include seafood and, to a lesser degree, dairy products.

Magnesium

The mineral magnesium is involved in hundreds of vital functions, including the liberation of energy from ATP, bone formation, muscle function, and the making of proteins. Aside from this, some research finds that magnesium may be of help to some diabetics and to those with *metabolic syndrome* because it improves insulin sensitivity.[101] Other studies hint that high doses of magnesium may modestly help lower blood pressure in people with hypertension.[102] Lower levels of magnesium appear to elevate C-reactive protein, a marker for heart disease.[103] Magnesium is found naturally in many products such as chocolate, green leafy vegetables, whole grains, nuts, and legumes. While obviously crucial for health, magnesium supplements may not be needed for healthy people. In high doses, a condition called *hypermagnesemia* can occur. Symptoms of hypermagnesemia include low blood pressure (hypotension), vomiting, and a slowing down of heart rate (bradycardia). These symptoms might begin to become evident when magnesium is used in excess of its upper tolerable intake limit of 350 mg per day.

Manganese

Manganese is a trace mineral that is involved in reproduction and the proper development of the nervous system. This mineral is also required for the production of *superoxide dismutase* (SOD), one of the body's natural antioxidants. Manganese synthase, a manganese-based enzyme, is also needed to make the non-essential amino acid glutamine. While known to be essential to humans since the 1930s, questions about manganese continue to arise. For example, some research hints that manganese may play a role in offsetting osteoporosis. Deficiencies in this mineral are not likely in the US, so supplements are usually not recommended for healthy adults. While manganese toxicity is unlikely to occur, animal and test tube studies suggest that it might result in the degeneration of the nervous system.[104] Manganese can also hinder the absorption of iron, which could contribute to anemia. Manganese supplements have no known exercise benefit. Foods that naturally contain manganese include shellfish, green leafy vegetables, berries, pineapple, teas, nuts, and whole grains.

Molybdenum

The trace mineral molybdenum assists a number of enzymes that help metabolize amino acids. Animal studies suggest that lack of this mineral might impact reproduction, decrease food consumption to unhealthy levels, and shorten lifespan. Deficiencies in molybdenum are very unlikely in healthy people, and too much molybdenum might interfere with copper absorption. While some research hints that molybdenum-deficient soil might be related to increased esophageal cancer, there is no good proof that molybdenum supplements prevent any form of cancer in humans. Most health experts recommend obtaining molybdenum from food and not supplements. Foods that naturally contain molybdenum include legumes, peas, milk, nuts, and grains.

Phosphorus

Phosphorous is needed by every cell of the body. When delving into studies on phosphorus, one quickly encounters the word "phosphate." Phosphate and phosphorus are essentially the same, as most of the body's phosphorus occurring in the form of phosphate. Readers are probably familiar with the energy molecules adenosine triphosphate (ATP) and creatine phosphate (CP), which both require phosphorus to function. Furthermore, both teeth and bones need phosphorus to harden, so a lack of this nutrient can weaken bones. While a deficiency in phosphorus is unlikely to occur in those eating a healthy diet, low levels of this nutrient can result in muscle weakness, an altered heartbeat, and decreased immunity.

For years, rumors have circulated that soft drinks and other phosphorus-containing beverages might deplete the body of calcium and contribute to osteoporosis. The reason for this speculation is that high phosphorus intake might stimulate parathyroid hormone (PTH), which, in turn, removes calcium from bones and could make bones weaker over time. While this makes sense in theory, such effects have only been observed under laboratory conditions in which people were put on a high-phosphorus/low-calcium diet.[105] A simpler reason for this trend might be that soda replaces milk and other calcium-rich foods from the diet. Other research finds that when calcium intake is high (2000 mg/day), high phosphorus intake does not appear to affect bone mineral density.[105] Foods that naturally contain phosphorus include milk, yogurt, and other dairy products. Meats are also a good source of this mineral.

Potassium

All life on earth is, in part, made possible because of potassium. Potassium, along with sodium, is indispensable for all muscle contraction as well as for the transmission of nerve impulses. This transmission of electrical signals is the reason why potassium and sodium are also referred to as electrolytes. A lack of potassium (or an increase in potassium excretion, which occurs in the case of vomiting or with the use of diuretics) can produce a condition called *hypokalemia* and can result in muscle weakness, general fatigue, altered heart function, cramping, and abdominal pain.

One of the significant areas of investigation with regard to potassium is blood pressure. Several studies have noted lower blood pressures in those with higher potassium intakes. Because fruits and vegetables contain potassium, these foods are often recommended to people with hypertension. In addition, fruits and vegetables are low in calories, which can lead to weight loss. Reduction in weight is also sometimes associated with reduced blood pressure.[106]

Bananas are a commonly-recognized potassium-containing food, with one medium-sized banana providing over 400 mg of this nutrient. However, bananas do not necessarily contain any more potassium than other healthy foods. For example, a medium-sized baked potato supplies over 700 mg of potassium. Other foods that naturally contain potassium include fruits and vegetables, nuts, fish, and beans.

Selenium

The trace mineral selenium appears to be essential to human health in a number of ways. For example, selenium is important to the immune system and is also required for the production of an intracellular antioxidant called glutathione peroxidase, which helps keep free radicals from getting out of hand. Selenium may show up in supplements alongside vitamin E because research finds that these two nutrients work synergistically. Other research suggests that selenium may be of help in reducing the risk of prostate cancer in men. That being said, the usefulness of selenium supplements is controversial and is usually not recommended for healthy people. Like many nutrients, small amounts of selenium appear to be helpful, but too much selenium (above the UL) has the potential to cause symptoms such as hair loss, fatigue, and a garlic-like odor of the breath.[107] Foods that naturally contain selenium include meats, seafood, and poultry.

Sodium

Sodium is one of the body's electrolytes and is partially responsible for the conduction of electrical nerve impulses. Thus, sodium is indispensable not only for nerve signal transmission, but for all muscle contractions (including the heart) as well. Too much sodium, however, is associated with high blood pressure (hypertension).

High blood pressure is defined as a consistent resting blood pressure of greater than or equal to 140/90 mm Hg. Over time, increased resting blood pressure can damage organs and accelerate heart disease. Besides hypertension, excessive sodium consumption is also one of the lifestyle behaviors associated with osteoporosis.

Sodium is found in many foods and is usually added to processed foods. As a general rule, anything that comes in a box or a can probably has some sodium added to it.

Besides table salt (sodium chloride), which comprises most of our sodium intake, sodium is also found in soy sauce, monosodium glutamate (MSG), baking powder, sodium saccharin, ketchup, onion salt, garlic salt, and some bottled mineral waters. Sea salt is often thought of as being healthy, but it has just as much sodium as table salt and may be a problem for those with hypertension.

Some foods are eligible to list certain health claims on their labels if they meet official standards. For example, foods may be listed as "sodium free" if they contain extremely small amounts of sodium (less than 5 mg per serving). Moreover, foods are said to be "reduced sodium" if they have 25% less sodium than that contained in the original version. Lastly, foods are considered "low sodium" if they have 140 mg or less sodium per serving. Though there is no RDA for sodium, people are usually advised to use 1500–2300 mg of sodium per day.

Zinc

Zinc is the second most plentiful trace mineral in the body, participating in hundreds of chemical reactions associated with proper immune function, the sense of smell and taste, wound healing, and reproduction to list just a few. Signs of zinc deficiency can include hair loss, dry skin, vision problems, low sperm count, low testosterone levels, as well as slowed growth and development.

One of the most popular topics of discussion when it comes to zinc is its impact on immunity. While the studies are controversial in that not all of them show that zinc helps, some research finds that zinc gluconate used every few hours beginning at the onset of a cold may help shorten the duration of symptoms by a few days.[109] Zinc appears to help the immune system battle colds by interfering with the replication of cold viruses. In other words, by limiting the spread of cold viruses, zinc may help give the immune system more time to mount an effective counter attack. Zinc supplements, however do not seem to boost immunity in people who are not sick. In fact, chronic use of zinc supplements might actually weaken the immune system![110]

With respect to exercise, some strength trainers and bodybuilders may supplement with zinc because a lack of this mineral has been shown to reduce testosterone levels in men.[108] The effect of zinc supplements on athletic ability, strength, and power, however, has not been adequately studied and many questions remain. Before supplementing with zinc, athletes should first determine whether they are currently ingesting enough of for this mineral. Zinc is found in many foods and may also be in other supplements commonly used by athletes. Foods that are good sources of zinc include oysters, fortified breakfast cereals, beef, and turkey.

The Major Minerals

Mineral	Dietary Sources	Major Functions	Deficiency	Signs of Excess
Calcium	Milk, cheese, yogurt, dark green vegetables	Blood clotting, nerve transmission, bone strength	Osteoporosis, stunted growth	None reported in humans
Phosphorous	Milk, cheese, meat, fish	Structural component of bone, teeth, cell membranes, ATP	Bone loss. Deficiency is rare	Possible calcium loss from bones
Potassium	Cantaloupe, potatoes, bananas, milk, meat	Nerve transmission, muscle contraction	Muscle cramps, irregular heart rhythm	Abnormal heart rhythm
Sulfur	Meats, milk, cheese	Helps with protein synthesis	Deficiency is rare	Very rare. Excess is excreted in urine and feces
Sodium	Table salt	Nerve transmission, muscle contraction	Muscle atrophy, nausea, weight loss	High blood pressure
Chlorine	Fruits, vegetables, salt-containing food	Helps maintain pH of body	Unlikely to occur if chloride-containing foods are consumed	High blood pressure
Magnesium	Green leafy vegetables, coffee, tea	Muscle contraction, extraction of energy from ATP	Growth problems	Depression, nausea, diarrhea

The Trace Minerals

Mineral	Dietary Sources	Major Functions	Deficiency	Signs of Excess
Iron	Lean meats, green leafy vegetables	Oxygen transport	Weakness, fatigue, infections	Iron overload disease
Fluorine	Drinking water, seafood	Helps with bone formation	Increased cavities	Nausea, vomiting, abnormal heart rhythm, death
Zinc	Meats, wheat germ	Protein synthesis	Growth problems	Fever, vomiting, diarrhea
Copper	Meats, drinking water	Needed for iron use	Anemia	Nausea, vomiting, diarrhea
Selenium	Seafood, meats, grains	DNA repair, immune functioning	Anemia	Hair and nail loss, nausea, vomiting
Iodine	Vegetables, iodized salt	Component of thyroid hormone	None reported in humans	Very high intakes inhibit thyroid activity
Chromium	Meats, nuts, cheese, whole grain bread	Involved in glucose and energy metabolism	Decreased ability to use glucose effectively	Some evidence that chromium (chromium picolinate) may cause DNA damage

Recommended Vitamin and Mineral Intakes

Vitamin	Adult RDA	Adult AI	Adult UL
Vitamin A	Men:600 µ Women: 700 µ		10,000 IU (3,000 µ)
Vitamin D	1 to 70: 600 IU. Over 70: 800 IU		2000 IU
Vitamin E	22 IU natural vitamin E or 33 IU synthetic vitamin E		100 IU synthetic / 1500 IU natural
Vitamin K		Men: 120 µ Women: 90 µ	Not established
Vitamin C	Men: 90 mg Women: 75 mg		2000 mg
Thiamin (B-1)	Men: 1.2 mg Women:1.1 mg		Not established
Riboflavin (B-2)	Men: 1.3 mg Women: 1.1 mg		Not established
Niacin (B-3)	Men 16 mg Women 14 mg		35 mg
Pantothenic Acid (B-5)		5 mg	Not established
Pyridoxine (B-6)	Men: up to age 50: 1.3 mg Men over age 50: 1.7 mg Women: to age 50: 1.3 mg Women over 50: 1.5 mg		100 mg
Folate (vitamin B9)	400 µ		1000 µ
Cyanocobalamin (B-12)	2.4 µ		Not established
Biotin	30 µ		Not established
Minerals	**Adult RDA**	**Adult AI**	**Adult UL**
Boron	Not established		20 mg
Calcium	To age 50: 1000 mg Over age 50: 1200 mg		2500 mg
Chromium	Men to age 50: 35 µ Men over 50: 30 µ Women to age 50: 25 µ Women over 50: 20 µ		Not established
Copper	900 µ		10 mg
Iodine	150 µ		1.1 mg
Iron	Men: 8 mg Women up to age 50: 18 mg Women over age 50: 8 mg		45 mg
Magnesium	Men to age 30: 400 mg Men over 30: 420 mg Women to age 30: 310 mg Women over 30: 320 mg		350 mg
Manganese		Men:2.3 mg Women: 1.8 mg	11 mg
Molybdenum	45 µ		2 mg
Phosphorus	700 mg		Up to age 70: 4,000 mg Over age 70: 3,000 mg
Potassium	Not established	4.7 g	
Selenium	55 µ		400 µ
Sodium	Not established		2300 mg
Zinc	Men: 11 mg Women: 8 mg		40 mg

As can be seen from the table, there is no RDA for some nutrients. For example, an RDA has not been established for potassium, but nutrition experts generally recommend 3000–3500 mg of this mineral be consumed in food each day.[93] Boron, once popular among some fitness enthusiasts because of the mistaken belief that it could raise testosterone levels, also has no RDA.

What Are Phytonutrients?

The prefix *phyto*- means "plant." *Phytonutrients* are not vitamins or minerals, but are components of fruits, vegetables, grains, and teas thought to play a role in health. Currently there is no RDA for phytonutrients and no known deficiency syndromes associated with a lack of these compounds. Emerging evidence, however, is finding that phytonutrients (phytochemicals) may play a role in health by preventing various diseases. For example, some evidence suggests that various phytonutrients may act as antioxidants and may protect the body from syndromes such as cancer and heart disease.

Examples of phytonutrients include the *carotenoids*, *anthocyanins*, and *isoflavonoids*, to name a few, though hundreds of phytonutrients are currently known to exist. Studies show that people who consume a diet rich in fruits and vegetables tend to be healthier overall than those who do not. These observations have prompted research designed to uncover which nutrients might be responsible for food's protective effects. Unfortunately, the research on phytonutrients is still in its infancy. For example, as mentioned previously, studies have found that smokers who use beta-carotene supplements have a *higher* rate of lung cancer compared to non-smokers.[80] This is just the opposite as is observed when people eat foods containing beta-carotene. Lycopene, a phytonutrient found in tomatoes, is sometimes used by men because of research hinting that it may help reduce one's risk for prostate cancer. However, most research on this nutrient involves eating tomatoes, not taking them in supplement form. It is possible that fruits, vegetables, grains, and teas protect against disease because of the interaction of thousands of phytonutrients working in concert with each other. If this is true, then consuming large amounts of single phytonutrients, like lycopene or beta carotene, might not be as beneficial as consuming fruits and vegetables—and may result in outcomes quite different than desired.

Nutrition Terminology

When discussing vitamins, minerals, and nutrition in general, readers encounter several terms and acronyms that bear discussing here:

International Units (IU). Some drugs and vitamins are measured not in milligrams or grams, but rather in international units. For example, the potency of vitamin E is often listed in international units (e.g., 400 IU). Confusion often arises when people try to convert between IUs and a more common unit of measure such as milligrams. International Units are a measure of the potency of a vitamin or drug, while milligrams, grams, and other units are measures of weight. Conversion factors do exist to help nutritionists translate IUs to milligrams, which may be necessary in certain clinical situations. For example, to convert from IUs to mg of dl alpha tocopherol (synthetic vitamin E), multiply the IUs by 0.45.

GRAS. The letters GRAS stand for *generally recognized as safe*, a term used by the FDA and other nutrition agencies to denote compounds that have been in the food supply before 1958. Thus substances listed as GRAS either have a long track record of safety or have scientific evidence affirming that they are safe for human consumption. Nutrition research is always continuing. By law, compounds that are currently listed as GRAS may in fact be de-listed as evidence contrary to their safety comes to light.

Bioavailability. This term refers to how much of a nutrient is available to be absorbed by the body. Some nutrients, like protein are highly absorbable, while others, like the mineral chromium, are less well absorbed.

Daily Value (DV). Daily values are listed on food labels and are based on the RDA. They represent the suggested nutrient intake levels that all persons can use, regardless of age or gender. The Daily Values, however, are based on a 2,000-calorie-per-day diet. As a rule, a healthy 2,000-calorie-per-day diet should provide daily values of 1,200 calories from carbohydrate, 600 calories from fat, and 25 grams of fiber.

Recommend Dietary Allowance (RDA). The RDA is the average daily intake of a nutrient that is sufficient to meet the needs of most healthy persons of a particular age and gender. There are many RDAs, including recommendations for children, adults, and pregnant women. In an attempt to make the RDA more applicable to all people, a set of terms was created bring all recommendations under the heading of "Dietary Reference Intakes" (DRI), which are defined below.

Dietary Reference Intake (DRI). This is a phrase with which many people may be unfamiliar, as it is used mostly in academic settings. The dietary reference intake is designed to be more all-encompassing than the RDA. In fact, DRIs actually contain the recommended dietary allowance. There are four DRI values:

1. **RDA:** The recommended dietary allowance mentioned above.

2. **Estimated Average Requirement (EAR).** This value is the amount used to meet the nutrient needs of half of healthy persons within a particular age and gender group. The EAR is one of the numbers that helps with the establishment of an RDA.

3. **Adequate Intake (AI).** For some nutrients, an RDA has not yet been determined. When no RDA is available, a nutrient is assigned an Average Intake (AI) number. These values are approximations of how much of a

nutrient is thought to be adequate for healthy individuals.

4. **Upper Tolerable Limit (UL)**. Too much of any nutrient might produce undesirable side effects. The Upper Tolerable Limit (UL) is the uppermost amount of a nutrient that can usually be tolerated by people without side effects. Intake that exceeds a nutrient's UL enhances the chances that side effects might occur. This is not to say that side effects will definitely occur, but that the *potential* for side effects is increased at levels above the UL.

Chapter 7

Dietary Supplements

Those in the fitness and nutrition field will undoubtedly be asked about dietary supplements at some point in their career. Currently, tens of thousands of dietary supplements are on the US market. While it is beyond the scope of this book to review all supplements, this chapter provides a basic review of some of those about which the fitness professional may be asked. For expanded reviews of these topics and over 100 other popular supplements, read my book *Nutritional Supplements: What Works and Why,* available at www.Joe-Cannon.com. Also see my website, Supplement-Geek.com.

What Are Dietary Supplements?

Dietary supplements refer to a wide range of substances that are meant to supplement a healthy diet. The official definition of the term "dietary supplement" stems from the Dietary Supplement Health and Education Act of 1994 (called *DSHEA* for short). According to this act, a dietary supplement is defined as:

> "a product (other than tobacco) intended to supplement the diet that bears or contains one or more of the following dietary ingredients: a vitamin, mineral, amino acid, herb, or other botanical OR a dietary substance used to supplement the diet by increasing the total dietary intake OR a concentrate, metabolite, constituent, extract, or combination of any ingredient described above AND intended for ingestion in the form of a capsule, powder, softgel, or gelcap, and not represented as a conventional food or as a sole item of a meal or the diet AND is labeled a dietary supplement."

This definition is the basis for all of the tens of thousands of supplements on the US market today. All dietary supplements sold in the United States must adhere to these guidelines. Products that fail to meet the criteria outlined in this definition cannot be legally called a "dietary supplement."

Occasionally, the Food and Drug Administration (FDA) takes action against companies marketing products that either do not adhere to DSHEA's supplement definition or that make specific claims that the product may act in a manner similar to a drug, which is illegal under current US law. Sometimes this action takes the form of a warning letter cautioning a company to curtail what the FDA deems an inappropriate marketing practice (like making drug claims). In other instances, the FDA may actually seize a product and ban its sale because of evidence that the product is inappropriately packaged, is adulterated with other substances, or is dangerous. Sometimes these actions scare people into thinking that the government is trying to restrict the sale of supplements. Indeed, editorials occasionally appear in some newspapers and magazines alleging that this is so. The odds of this happening, however, are quite low. The DSHEA has been the "law of the land" since 1994. In addition, evidence continues to accumulate that some supplements, when used properly, have beneficial effects on health.

What Is Peer-Reviewed Research?

Peer-reviewed research is the best type of study. To have a study peer-reviewed means that, before the study was published in a scientific journal, it was first reviewed by other competent scientists ("peers") whose job is to look for mistakes or flaws in the experiment. Any errors in research discovered during the peer review process must be fixed before the study is accepted for publication. Essentially, having a peer-reviewed study published means that you did your homework, dotted all of your "i's," and crossed all of your "t's." The scientific journals in which peer-reviewed research is published are generally not found in the magazine section of your local supermarket. You must subscribe to them, and subscriptions may cost hundreds of dollars per year! Articles appearing in popular magazines are generally not peer-reviewed, but they sometimes are based on peer-reviewed research studies.

Examples of peer-reviewed scientific journals:

- *Journal of Nutrition*
- *Pharmacotherapy*
- *International Journal of Sports Nutrition and Exercise Metabolism*
- *Medicine and Science in Sports and Exercise*
- *Journal of Strength and Conditioning Research*

Amino Acid Supplements

Amino acids are often called the building blocks of proteins because many amino acids linked together form proteins. Some people take amino acids supplements in order to enhance muscular strength and development or to help with recovery. While consumption of amino acids may, indeed, contribute to muscle growth, supplements that contain amino acids may not be the best course of action. There is no guarantee that amino acids in an ingested supplement will be used to help build muscle. The body may incorporate the amino acids from the supplement into growing muscles, or it could simply use them to make earwax! Another problem with taking just one or a few amino acids is that this practice does not provide the same broad spectrum of amino acids as food offers. Amino acid supplements also tend to be more expensive than food.

Amino acids do have different properties, and research hints that some of them may have usefulness that goes beyond their incorporation into muscle proteins. For example, marathon runners may use supplements that only contain branch chain amino acids (BCAA). These amino acids—specifically leucine, isoleucine, and valine—are thought to compete with and maybe impede the entry of tryptophan (another amino acid) into the brain. The body needs tryptophan to make serotonin, which is associated with fatigue. By reducing tryptophan via BCAA supplements, runners might, in theory, stave off fatigue during exercise. BCAAs may also reduce the body's reliance on glycogen during exercise and thus extend the time before glycogen exhaustion sets in. Currently, however, the effectiveness of this strategy is questionable, as research has found that it may or may not help. Some evidence hints that BCAAs may stimulate the release of insulin from the beta cells of the pancreas.[111] As such, BCAA supplements might interact with medications used by diabetics. For athletes who are considering BCAA supplements but who are on a budget, it may be helpful to remember that 3 ounces of tuna fish supplies the body with ample supply of these amino acids. Thus, supplementation may not be necessary.

Androstenedione

Androstenedione ("andro") is not really a dietary supplement, but rather a hormone made within the adrenal glands.[20] Andro is sometimes popular among strength trainers because it is one chemical step from the anabolic hormone testosterone. Thus, the rationale behind using androstenedione is that it will lead to higher testosterone levels, which, in turn, might promote enhanced muscular development. However, clinical studies to date have failed to show that androstenedione enhances muscular growth, strength, or athletic performance.[8, 43] In fact, some research finds that it may raise estrogen levels in men! Because it is a hormone, androstenedione is not without risks. Emerging evidence suggests that androstenedione may lower HDL (good cholesterol) levels, which may raise the risk for heart disease. Pro-hormones such as androstenedione should be used with caution because of a lack of proof regarding their long-term safety.

Black Cohosh

Black cohosh is an herb that grows in North America and was first introduced to early European settlers by the Native American Indians. These days, the main purpose for which people use black cohosh is to relieve menopause symptoms. The scientific names for black cohosh are *Actaea racemosa* and *Cimicifuga racemosa*.

Some studies have found that black cohosh may be of modest help in reducing hot flashes and other symptoms associated with menopause and premenstrual syndrome (PMS). However, not all research finds that it works. In addition, most studies finding positive results with black cohosh agree that at least a few weeks of continued use is needed before any reduction in menopausal symptoms is noticed. Because of its apparent ability to reduce some symptoms of menopause, it has generally been believed that black cohosh has estrogen-like properties. However, this is still being investigated, and debate continues as to how black cohosh works.

Osteoporosis is a disease in which bones become brittle and break easily. Estrogen is needed to help keep bones strong. Because black cohosh is thought to possess estrogen-like qualities, some feel that this herb may help reduce one's risk for osteoporosis. Currently, this is pure speculation, and black cohosh should not be used as a substitute in place of osteoporosis medications prescribed by a physician.

Carnitine

Carnitine (also called L carnitine) is sometimes popular among those trying to lose weight. Carnitine is one of the molecules involved in moving fat to the mitochondria to be broken down (burned) for energy. Because of this, some speculate that additional dietary carnitine may help the fat-burning process by bringing even more fat than normally possible to the mitochondria to be utilized. While this might sound plausible in theory, most of the research on carnitine supplements to date finds that this is not the case.[13, 57]

Chromium Picolinate

Chromium is a trace mineral. *Picolinate acid* (which is part of chromium picolinate) is a natural metabolite of the amino acid tryptophan. One of the roles of chromium is to help regulate blood sugar.[26] Studies of young, growing animals have hinted that chromium picolinate may be effective for reducing body fat as well as for improving muscle mass. However, many human studies have failed to show this effect.[60] Other investigations of chromium ranging from college football players to overweight military personal have found neither reductions in body fat nor enhancements in muscle mass following chromium supplementation.[36] Based upon the preponderance of current evidence, chromium picolinate does not appear to contribute significantly to muscular development or fat loss in healthy humans.

Creatine

Creatine is a natural product made in the body and is also found in meats and fish. Studies dating back to the 1960s have found that the use of creatine supplements may improve strength and power. As such, creatine is sold as a dietary supplement touted to improve strength and power in those participating in very high intensity activities like powerlifting, bodybuilding, and sprinting.[60] When ingested, creatine becomes *phosphocreatine*, a molecule that regenerates ATP during times when ATP must be made extremely quickly. As such, creatine acts like a supercharger for ATP production. Faster energy production rates translate into an ability to sustain high intensity activity for a longer period of time and an enhanced capacity to recuperate between bouts of exercise. These characteristics allow an athlete to sustain a high-intensity stimulus for a longer period of time, which stimulates the body to make more muscle proteins (myosin, actin, etc.) that help muscles become stronger. To phrase this in another way, the longer the muscles are under stress, the stronger they become.

Creatine is of little benefit to those participating in long-duration or low-intensity activities like jogging, triathlons, hiking, or yoga. Likewise, creatine supplements are probably of little help to those engaged in moderate-intensity resistance training programs. In other words, creatine would be of more help to those lifting a weight for 1–5 repetitions than to those who perform 12–20 reps.

Creatine and Sports

Creatine Might Help	
• Powerlifting	• Bodybuilding
• Football	• Shot putting
• Sprinting	• Javelin throwing
• Boxing	• Martial arts
Creatine Might Not Help	
• Triathlons	• Marathons
• Group aerobics classes	• Circuit strength training
• Horse racing	• Bicycling
• Jogging	• Hiking

Loading creatine—a practice in which people take a lot of creatine for the first week (typically 20–25 grams per day)—does not seem to be necessary or beneficial. Research shows that a month of using only 3 grams of creatine per day puts as much creatine in the muscles as does taking 20 grams in one week.[129]

With respect to side effects, no serious negative side effects have been observed with creatine to date. Rumors of abdominal cramping and muscle or tendon tears resulting from creatine supplementation are possible but have generally not been observed in research. The most consistent side effect from creatine supplementation is an increase in body weight, which is most likely due to increased water retention.[60] People with kidney problems are usually cautioned against using creatine for fear that it might overtax already wakened kidneys. Creatine might also be detrimental to those with liver problems. Many different creatine products are on the market. The type that has been used most commonly in research is *creatine monohydrate*.

Echinacea

Echinacea is generally regarded throughout the world as an herb capable of helping the body combat colds and other infections. Specifically, some research finds that echinacea may be able to reduce the duration and severity of colds by roughly 10–30% when taken at the very start of cold symptoms.

Three different species of echinacea are known to exist: *Echinacea angustifolia, Echinacea pallida,* and *Echinacea purpurea*. Of these, the latter species has been the most common subject of study. How echinacea stimulates the immune system is still a mystery, and the active ingredients in the plant are still under investigation. Also remaining in question is how much is needed. With respect to infections, one thing does seem clear—echinacea does not prevent colds when taken every day. In fact, regular use of this herb may actually depress the immune system![29]

In terms of side effects, because of its possible stimulation of immune system cells, echinacea is not recommended for those with autoimmune diseases such as rheumatoid arthritis, lupus, or type I diabetes. Likewise, the use of echinacea is controversial in those with HIV infection because it might worsen symptoms.[29] It is also noteworthy to mention that not all research shows that echinacea is effective for battling colds. Remember, all herbs are basically unrefined medicines. As such, they can interact with prescription medications that people may be taking and could, therefore, be dangerous.

Ephedra

Ephedrine is a drug derived from the plant *ephedra*, which mimics the action of adrenalin (epinephrine) in the body. Another popular name for ephedra is *Ma Huang*. Some studies have concluded that ephedrine use can promote small amounts of weight loss, probably an average of about 2 pounds more per week than without the use of ephedrine.[49] Because the amount of weight lost is small, ephedra is often combined with other agents such as caffeine and aspirin, which are said to boost its effects.[18]

Side effects from ephedrine use can include elevated blood pressure and heart rate, as well as strokes and seizures.[18] Psychosis has also been reported following the use of ephedrine.[18] Ephedra can raise blood sugar levels, so it may be inappropriate for diabetics. Because ephedrine can elevate heart rate and blood pressure, it is also not appropriate for those with heart or blood pressure disorders or for those with a family history of these diseases. At least 100 deaths associated with the use of ephedrine-containing products have been reported to the FDA, which is one reason it's been banned from being used in supplements.

Some supplements may contain other stimulants that "look like" ephedra. For example, bitter orange (*Citrus aurantium*) may be found in several weight loss supplements. Still other compounds include DMAA, DMBA higenamine. While several of these stimulant-like ingredients lack proof of their effectiveness, they it's possible that they may be accompanied by many of the same precautions as ephedra itself.

Glucosamine Sulfate

Glucosamine sulfate is a compound made naturally in the body and plays a role in the proper formation of cartilage.[19] Specifically, the sugar glucose and the amino acid glutamine unite to form glucosamine sulfate. Studies dating back to the 1970s have noted that glucosamine sulfate might help reduce the pain associated with osteoarthritis, the most common type of arthritis that occurs when the cartilage cushioning between bones wears away.[19] Because of this, glucosamine sulfate is a popular remedy among those seeking a natural alternative to arthritis drugs. Most glucosamine research generally finds that it helps about as much as aspirin and that it takes about 2 months before a reduction in pain is noticed. How glucosamine seems to work is not well understood, and some studies even show that it might not work. While glucosamine does not seem to restore joint cartilage, some evidence does hint that this supplement may help by slowing the progression of osteoarthritis.[116] It should be mentioned that the best evidence is for glucosamine sulfate. Many supplements contain another form called glycosamine HCL which appears to be less effective.

Glucosamine supplements are often combined with another compound called chondroitin sulfate. Whether or not glucosamine plus chondroitin work better than glucosamine alone is controversial. Men should ask their doctors about chondroitin sulfate. Some research hints that it may have an effect on prostate cancer. For more info on this, see my blog post "Chondroitin Sulfate And Prostate Cancer?" at Supplement-Geek.com.

With respect to side effects, glucosamine sulfate appears to be generally safe. Occasionally, questions as to whether glucosamine raises blood sugar levels surface, but this effect has not been well documented in humans. People using blood thinner medications should be cautious, however, as glucosamine and chondroitin may both interact with blood thinner medications.

Cleanse Supplements

Supplements that are said to "cleanse" the body are popular for weight loss. But do they work? The ingredients in many of these products actually are fiber. Since fiber is a laxative, its wise for trainers to remember that most cleanse supplements are also laxatives. The problem with laxatives for weight loss is that they work at the large intestine —where the *poop* is. Cleanses do not work at the small intestine —where we absorb food/calories from. Because of this, the weight that is lost through the use of cleanse supplements is mostly fecal matter and water. As such, they don't promote any real weight loss. Some cleanse supplements may contain an ingredient called *senna*, which comes from the senna plant. Senna is a laxative because it irritates large intestine causing the expulsion of fecal matter. A problem with cleanse supplements is that if they *work too well*, they can be dangerous. For example, diarrhea can lead to dehydration and depletion of electrolytes which can interfere with the way the heart beats.

Garcinia Cambogia

Garcinia cambogia, also called hydroxy citric acid (HCA) is an ingredient that may be found in weight loss supplements because of some research noting that it might lower appetite as well as reduce the transformation of carbs into fat. Some clinical trials have noted that garcinia may help people lose weight. Other studies however have not found it works. It's worth noting that studies showing that it worked also combined garcinia with eating fewer calories. Thus, taking garcinia cambogia supplements without also eating fewer calories may not work. Studies showing positive effects on weight loss generally used between 1.5-3 grams of garcinia per day. That may be more than is in some supplements. One drawback to most of the studies is that they generally didnt last long. Most only last 2-3 months for example. Thus, long term weight loss effects needs more research. At Supplement-Geek.com is a review titled "Garcinia Cambogia (HCA)

Review of Weight Loss Research" that goes into greater detail for those who want to know more.

Glucomannan

Glucomannan, also called Konjac root, is a fiber that expands when exposed to liquids. Because of this, it's found in some weight loss supplements and those marketed to diabetics. Some studies have noticed that glucomannan may help people lose weight and those which report positive outcomes have used between 1-3 grams per day. Glucomannan is different than another fiber called *Alpha Cyclodextrin* ("FBCX") which is thought to work by coating fat molecules, making them unable to be absorbed by the body. More research is needed on both fibers to better understand the roles they play in long term weight loss.

Supplements and the Fitness Professional

Despite advertisements to the contrary, the words "natural" and "safe" do not mean the same thing. Fitness professionals should investigate supplements for side effects, drug interactions, quality, and proof that substantiates a product's advertised claims before discussing them with clients. While there is little doubt that some dietary supplements may hold promise for improving health, wellbeing, and some aspects of exercise performance, they should never been viewed as a shortcut. All dietary supplements are designed to *supplement* a healthy diet—not to replace it. As always, good nutrition is the foundation for all exercise and wellness programs.

Before discussing any produce with clients, fitness trainers should also check with their employer. Some fitness facilities may strictly prohibit trainers from discussing supplements club members. It is also noteworthy to mention that some personal trainer liability insurance carriers will not protect fitness professionals from lawsuits brought about as a result of dietary supplements.

There is little doubt that personal trainers, group aerobics instructors, and other professionals in the fitness industry have been courted by the vitamin and supplement community as representatives to further market products to the public at large. On the surface, there is nothing wrong with this form of capitalism and networking, but fitness trainers must remember that their first duty is to their clients. Products that a health professional advocate reflect his or her beliefs and quality of service. Before discussing or recommending any dietary supplement, questions should always be asked. The questions listed below can be used as a guide to help when researching dietary supplements.

Dietary Supplements: Questions to Ask Yourself

1. Is there any published, peer-reviewed research showing that the product works?
2. If so, is the research on the product itself or on the ingredients found in the product?
3. Are the levels of ingredients in the product the same as those used in research?
4. On whom was the research conducted (men, women, bacteria, animals)?
5. If the product is promoted for weight loss, how was weight loss determined during research? Underwater weighing is the most accurate method available.
6. Is the research published as a full-fledged scientific paper (i.e., not an abstract)?
7. How many peer-reviewed studies on the product have been published that find that it does what it is reported to do?
8. Have any side effects or drug interactions been observed in research?
9. If the answer to question #8 is yes, what are the side effects and drug interactions?

Supplement Buzz Words

Advertisements for supplements tend to use a host of words to convey to the public that a product is of high quality. Popular buzz words used in advertisements include:

• Clinically proven	• Technology	• Modulate	• Anti-aging	• Miracle
• Patented	• Breakthrough	• Bioactive	• Quick	• Toxin
• Amazing	• All-natural	• Innovative	• Easy	• Cleanse

Words and phrases like these show up frequently in health, fitness, and nutrition advertisements. In reality, all of these terms are vaguely defined and, to the trained professional, mean very little. Remember that words like these should never take the place of quality, peer-reviewed research that has been published in clinical journals.

Because fitness trainers see people frequently, they often find themselves on the front lines when it comes to fielding questions regarding nutrition and supplements. I believe that what personal trainers need to remember most when discussing supplements is that client safety must be the top priority. If anything bad happened as a result of a recommendation, personal trainer liability insurance will probably not be of any help in the case of a lawsuit.

On my website, Joe-Cannon.com, you will find a blog post entitled, "Should Personal Trainers Recommend Supplements?" Every fitness trainer needs to read that post, because it presents information that most trainers have never been heard about before.

Chapter 8

Metabolism

It seems that everyone likes to talk about metabolism. Some people have "slow" metabolisms, while others have "fast" metabolisms. The problem is that few people understand what metabolism is. That is what this chapter is all about.

Right now as you read these words, millions of chemical reactions are occurring. Some of these chemical reactions result in something being created, while others undoubtedly break things down. Thus, metabolism may be defined as the sum total of all building-up and tearing-down processes in the body. The building-up metabolic processes are called *anabolism*. It is from the word anabolism that we get the term *anabolic*. The classic example of an anabolic reaction is the building of new muscle tissue, although the formation of new cells to line the digestive track is also anabolic. At the other end of the spectrum are the tearing-down metabolic processes, which are referred to as *catabolism*. It is from the word catabolism that the term *catabolic* is derived. In some circles, catabolism is given a negative connotation. This is understandable, especially given that the breakdown of muscle that occurs from disuse or disease is a catabolic reaction. It is important, however, for the fitness professional to recognize that not all catabolic reactions are bad. For example, the digestion of food is an essential catabolic reaction. Moreover, the breakdown of ATP, our ultimate energy molecule, and the breakdown of glycogen, our stored carbohydrate reserve, are also catabolic reactions.

Another way in which to understand metabolism is to define it as the number of calories consumed (burned) at rest. This definition gives rise to the terms *resting metabolic rate* and *basal metabolic rate*. Resting metabolic rate (or **RMR**) is the speed at which we burn calories in a resting state and accounts for approximately 70% of our daily caloric expenditure.[5] Basal metabolic rate (or **BMR**) is the minimum number of calories needed to keep us alive. You are at your basal metabolic rate when you are sleeping. While often used interchangeably, RMR and BMR are technically not the same thing—basal metabolic rate is lower than resting metabolic rate.

Factors that Impact Metabolism

It turns out that the rate at which we burn calories can be affected by several factors. As a general rule, men tend to have slightly higher metabolisms than women. Thus, gender is a factor that impacts metabolism. Other factors that influence metabolism include:

- **Age.** Metabolism tends to decrease as we grow older. Typically, resting metabolic rate drops by about 2–5% per decade after age 25.[27] This is one reasons why people tend to gain weight as they grow older.

- **Climate:** Metabolism tends to increase in colder environments. This makes sense, given that the body wants to maintain an internal temperature of about 98.6 degrees F. Lowering the outside temperature essentially makes the body fire up the furnace!

- **Thermic effect of food:** The thermic effect of food (TEF) refers to the fact that calories (energy) are required to digest and metabolize food. Thus, eating raises metabolism, though not very much. One reason why protein is sometimes used by those trying to lose weight is that it boosts metabolism more than carbohydrate or fat. This is because protein has a slightly higher thermic effect than the other two macronutrients.

- **Activity level:** Exercise can raise metabolism.

- **Hormones:** Hormones are chemical messengers. While thyroid hormone (thyroxin) plays a role in metabolism, so, too, do other hormones like testosterone, growth hormone, and insulin. Some hardcore bodybuilders may even inject insulin because it helps put sugar in cells and encourages the body to utilize amino acids. The problem, however, with non-diabetics injecting insulin is that, when injected, the body stops making its own insulin. Upon stopping insulin injections, the body may actually rebound into a diabetic state. Another problem is that no evidence demonstrates that the injection of insulin by non-diabetics improves muscle mass, strength, or athletic performance.

- **Body composition:** Muscle is a metabolically active tissue and consumes more calories at rest than fat. Muscle mass alone contributes to approximately 22% of one's RMR.[5] Thus, the more muscle a person has within his or her body, the greater his or her resting metabolic rate (RMR) tends to be. While the suggestion is controversial, some have estimated that every pound of muscle burns somewhere between 20 and 80 extra calories per day.

Exercise and Metabolism

One of the main reasons why people exercise when trying to lose weight is to boost metabolism. Exercise can be subdivided into aerobic and anaerobic activity. Both types are important, yet each impacts metabolic rate differently. For example, minute by minute, we tend to expend (burn) more calories during aerobic exercise than during resistance training. To illustrate, a 150-pound man burns approximately 648 calories per hour during aerobic exercise but only 432 calories per hour during strength training.[5]

Another way to differentiate between aerobic and anaerobic activity is by the length of time for which each elevates metabolism. Aerobic exercise has the most significant impact on metabolic rate during the activity itself. This can easily be seen from the example of the man given in the previous paragraph. However, metabolism tends to return to normal resting levels 1–2 hours after cessation of the activity.[133] Resistance training, on the other hand, may lead to elevations of metabolic rate lasting 16 or more hours after exercise.[5] That being said, not all research shows that resistance training significantly raises RMR.[133] Other factors that might also contribute to this post-strength training elevation in metabolic rate include the amount of muscle used during exercise, the weight or volume of weight lifted, the length of rest periods between sets, and the fitness level of the individual. Alterations in these variables may contribute to the conflicting results of exercise on RMR.

Dieting and Metabolism

Studies have shown that dieting can result in the lowering of both resting and basal metabolism.[36] In fact, severe calorie restriction may lower RMR by as much as 45%.[36] This reduction in metabolic rate actually makes sense when one considers that the body does not "understand" why less food is being eaten. As far as the body is concerned, a global catastrophe might have caused the reduction in food intake, but in reality, a convenience store may be located just down the street! The body only knows that fewer calories are being consumed, and it does the only thing that it can to stay alive—it slows the rate of fuel (calorie) consumption. In the event of a global catastrophe, a slower metabolic rate would mean that a person might live long enough to find more food. While staying alive in case of an emergency is obviously a good thing, the slowing of metabolism that accompanies dieting can sabotage one's weight loss progress by making it more difficult to lose weight. This is one of the reasons why most diets do not work in the long run.

Another problem with diet-induced reductions in metabolic rate is that the body may begin to begin to digest its own muscle tissue to stay alive. This could lead to the atrophy of muscle size and strength. As many fitness professionals are aware, when a muscle cell is lost, it never returns. Unfortunately, humans are not able to make new muscle cells— all that the body may do is build up muscle that remains.

Related to the more familiar type of atrophy described above is a process of which some fitness professionals are unaware—*sarcopenia*. **Sarcopenia**, an age-related loss of muscle tissue, tends to occur as we grow older and involves the loss of type II muscle cells. The body has two types of muscle cells—*type I* and *type II*. Type I (slow-twitch) fibers are used during endurance activities, while type II (fast-twitch) fibers are designed for strength and power. Type II fibers are divided into two categories. *Type IIa* fibers are fast-twitch muscle cells capable of exhibiting muscular endurance and generating a significant amount of strength. *Type IIb* muscle fibers are also fast-twitch fibers but are completely anaerobic muscle cells that produce far more strength and power than their counterpart. While sarcopenia normally occurs as one ages, long-term, low-calorie dieting, coupled with inadequate protein and nutrient intake, might accelerate this process. The reason for this is that the body, in an attempt to keep itself alive, performs a sort of "triage" to assess what may stay and what should be broken down to maintain life processes. Unfortunately, as we age, we tend to exercise less. Moreover, when we diet, energy levels may plummet so much that we may not be able to exercise regularly. In such instances, the body may begin to break down type IIb muscle fibers because it no longer believes that it needs them to survive. If left unchecked, this phenomenon would eventually have a detrimental impact on one's quality of life and ability to engage in physical activity.

Obviously, the process of sarcopenia described above is a worst-case scenario. For most healthy people, a few weeks of dieting is unlikely to cause a detrimental condition such as sarcopenia. For fitness professionals working with older adults, however, sarcopenia is a real possibility. Older adults tend to eat less food, especially in the form of protein. They also tend to exercise less than younger individuals. Of those older adults who do exercise, very few strength train. While the process that leads to sarcopenia remains somewhat mysterious, it appears that two of the best practices through which we may reduce its impact are eating well and exercising regularly.

Estimating Metabolic Rate

There are several ways to estimate metabolic rate. One popular method involves multiplying the body weight of males by 11 and that of women by 10. [27]

| Males | RMR = Body weight X 11 cal/lb |
| Females | RMR = Body weight X 10 cal/lb |

The numbers 10 and 11 are used because it is estimated that a man's body needs about 11 calories per pound to maintain its basic operational needs, while a woman's body needs about 10 calories per pound. For example, a 200-pound man needs about 200 x 11 = 2,200 calories per day to maintain resting metabolic rate. A 200-pound woman needs about 200 x 10 = 2,000 calories a day. This method, however, is not highly accurate, as it only estimates *resting* metabolic rate. What if you do more than "rest?" After all, people typically ask about metabolism because they want to lose weight, so they are likely to engage in some physical activity. These equations don't factor in exercise and other daily activities.

Another equation is to multiply one's desired body weight by 13. For example, if one were 160 pounds and wanted to be 140 pounds, 140 x 13 = 1,820 calories. In theory, eating 1,820 calories in this example should help one to eventualy reach his or her 140-pound goal. Still another basic way to reach this goal is to simply reduce the number of calories that one eats. Generally, eating 250–300 fewer calories per day promotes weight loss in most people. Fitness professionals should be conscious not to decrease calorie intake too much, lest they significantly decrease metabolic rate and negatively impact weight-loss progress. According to some, consistently losing more than ½ pound per week might lower metabolic rate.

Chapter 9

Eating Disorders

Fitness professionals will undoubtedly come across people who have issues with eating. This is especially true for those counseling clients about nutrition. While this chapter is not all encompassing, its main goals are to review some of the most common conditions and to provide insights into assisting individuals in coping with these problems. Eating disorders are serious conditions and, when taken to extremes, can be fatal. The fitness professional should never view him- or herself as a client's only resource, but should instead seek out other competent professionals within the healthcare continuum (i.e., registered dietitians, psychologists, and physicians) when faced with issues beyond his or her scope of practice.

Female Athletic Triad

Female athletic triad is a phrase coined by the American College of Sports Medicine (ACSM) to describe a syndrome of three distinct but often related medical disorders frequently observed in adolescent and young adult female athletes. The syndromes comprising female athletic triad are:[3]

1. Disordered eating patterns
2. Amenorrhea
3. Osteoporosis

These three issues are of growing concern, especially due to the pressure placed on adolescent girls to maintain what they think is an "ideal" body weight. In women who develop female athletic triad, excessive exercise or inadequate nutrition affect the ovaries, which respond by reducing estrogen output. Reduced estrogen levels, in turn, cause bone loss and accelerate the development of osteoporosis. This can have a profoundly detrimental impact on quality (and quantity) of life years later.

Estrogen also plays a role in protecting women from heart disease. Thus, an issue not often mentioned is that a lack of estrogen due to amenorrhea might also increase the risk of heart attack in younger women. Amenorrhea may also affect cardiovascular health years after women's sports careers are over. The consequences of amenorrhea may not be taken seriously by young athletes who think of themselves as invincible and do not comprehend its possible far reaching consequences. In fact, fitness professionals should not be surprised when competitive athletic women are not overly concerned with their lack of menstruation. Amenorrhea, however, is a serious condition, and women experiencing symptoms of this disorder should be referred to a physician or gynecologist equipped to monitor them over time.

Who Is at Risk for Female Athletic Triad?

Women who participate in sports and who strive for thinness in order to perform better or to look better while performing are at risk for female athletic triad. These women tend to be overly concerned with weight, food, and body shape. Athletes in whom female athletic triad may be observed include but are not limited to gymnasts, jockeys, swimmers, race car drivers, female professional wrestlers, bodybuilders, fashion models, marathon runners, and triathletes. Female athletic triad may also be common in college female athletes whose education is partially or fully funded through athletic scholarships. It is important to note that it is not only elite athletic females who may develop this condition. Any physically active female may be at risk of developing female athletic triad.[3]

Dealing with Female Athletic Triad

While there are no easy answers, fitness professionals working with young athletic females should strive to instill in their clients a healthy body image. Negative comments about body weight should be avoided. Coaches who instill a negative body image in a female athlete as a way of coaxing her to lose weight have the potential to harm the woman's health for years to come.

Currently, the incidence of female athletic triad is not fully known. However, studies suggest that anywhere from 15–62% of female athletes have some form of disordered eating.[21] Given these statistics, young girls should be encouraged not to be influenced by what the media depicts as the "perfect body." After all, what the media often depicts as "healthy" is often unrealistic and is achieved through airbrushing and other camera tricks. The young female should also feel comfortable enough to communicate her feelings to both her parents and her physician. While often viewed as a touchy issue, menstrual cycle patterns may be crucial for identifying those with this condition. The intervention of a registered dietician or sports nutritionist who has experience with female athletic triad may be necessary to help the athlete get back on track.

Anorexia Nervosa

Anorexia nervosa is the refusal to maintain an appropriate body weight for one's age, height, and gender. Individuals with anorexia nervosa have an intense fear of gaining weight and a preoccupation with dieting and being thin.[36] Basically, people with this condition do not eat very much. In spite of being thin, people with anorexia nervosa view themselves as being overweight. To combat the perceived "fatness," individuals often subject themselves to large volumes of exercise. With weight loss comes the eventual stopping of menstruation (amenorrhea) described previously. While anorexia nervosa is present in between 1–2% of the general population of America, between 6–20% of those afflicted with the syndrome die as a result of various factors including suicide, heart disease, and infections. [36]

An aspect of this condition not often addressed is oral health. On the surface, the health of the gums, teeth, and oral cavity may seem trivial when compared to the other outcomes described above, but the preservation of a healthy mouth is nonetheless an essential aspect of long-term health maintenance. Here is why: Research has linked gum disease and tooth decay to the development of heart disease. Some evidence suggests that people with gum disease have higher levels of C reactive protein (CRP), a compound that appears to impact the risk of heart disease. Thus, a lack of proper nutrition, coupled with an intake of nutrient deficient foods, might not only lead to bone loss and gum disease, but may increase heart disease risk as well.

Signs and Symptoms of Anorexia Nervosa

- Refusal to maintain appropriate body weight for one's gender, age, and size
- Extreme fear of gaining weight in spite of being very underweight
- Altered body image (i.e., the perception of being fat even though one is underweight for one's age, gender, and height)
- The absence of at least three consecutive menstrual cycles

Bulimia Nervosa

The name *bulimia nervosa* makes reference to the almost insatiable appetite observed in those afflicted with the syndrome.[36] Bulimia is characterized by frequent occurrences of binge eating (usually at night), which is almost always followed by vomiting.[36] Bulimia is a somewhat more frequent manifestation of disordered eating than anorexia nervosa, as bulimia is seen in 2–4% of adolescents and adults. The majority of individuals afflicted with this syndrome are female.[36] Following binge eating, individuals with bulimia tend to starve themselves by fasting and may also use laxatives or water pills to aid in the expulsion of ingested food.[36] Individuals with bulimia may also exercise excessively as a way to rid themselves of calories. Bulimia may occur in those who are overweight or of normal weight.

Signs and Symptoms of Bulimia Nervosa

- Excessive concern with body weight and body composition
- Frequent gains and losses in weight
- Visits to the bathroom following meals
- Recurrent instances of binge eating, usually in secret
- Binge eating followed by periods of not eating and/or vomiting
- The use of laxatives or water pills to expel food, or the use of excessive exercise to expend calories
- Irregular menstrual cycles

Muscle Dysmorphia

Women usually figure prominently in most discussions on eating disorders and body image problems, while men often remain neglected. This is unfortunate, for men can suffer from these concerns as well. Although not technically classified as an eating disorder, one example of a little known eating issue frequently observed in men is *muscle dysmorphia*. Sometimes the term muscle dysmorphia is used interchangeably with the more popular "Adonis Syndrome," but technically, they are not the same. Adonis Syndrome can refer to a number of body image or physical conditions that men may want to change or take steps to avoid. These conditions can range from hair loss to plastic surgery, sexual potency issues, and body fat reduction, among others. Muscle dysmorphia, however, is specific in its reference to the intense desire to have bigger muscles. Symptoms of muscle dysmorphia may include excessive exercise (sometimes exceeding 2 hours per day) that takes priority over other activities such as keeping a job, spending time with family, and engaging in hobbies; avoidance of social situations; and a preoccupation with how attractive one's body looks. Those with muscle dysmorphia may also experiment with steroids or dietary supplements reputed to increase muscle size and strength. Essentially, men with muscle dysmorphia see themselves as small and weak even though they appear big and strong to everyone else. Some individuals with muscle dysmorphia may have eating disorders (about 30%), experience anxiety and depression over their body image, and may take part in radical diets. In this respect, muscle dysmorphia shares some characteristics with anorexia, which was described previously. In fact, muscle dysmorphia used to be called "reverse anorexia" in some medical circles.[122] Men experiencing muscle dysmorphia may also wear layers of clothing to look bigger or to cover up their perceived smallness. Injuries resulting from overtraining syndrome may also appear in these individuals. While this condition may occur in any sport, it appears most common in sports like bodybuilding, in which muscle symmetry is emphasized.

Symptoms like those described above are general and could probably describe a number of people, including even some fitness professionals. By themselves, some of these signs may be perfectly normal. However, when combined with depression, steroid abuse, low self-esteem, anxiety, and/or suicidal thoughts, or when one's preoccupation with exercising to improve appearance is at the expense of family, friends, and occupation, then counseling with a qualified professional may be in order.

Signs and Symptoms of Muscle Dysmorphia

- Preoccupation with bodily appearance
- Excessive time spent working out
- Exercising at the expense of family, friends, and hobbies
- Inaccurate perception of being small or weak
- Continuation of exercise even when injured
- Layering of clothing to appear bigger
- Steroid abuse

Chapter 10

Client Assessment

For many fitness professionals, especially those who are new to the field, the question of what needs to be done when first meeting with a new client can be overwhelming. Most fitness professionals have a working understanding of weight lifting technique, target heart rate, calories, protein, fat, carbohydrate, and related issues, but deciding what needs to be completed before an effective exercise and nutrition program is designed can be perplexing. This chapter deals with issues surrounding how to assess the current fitness and nutrition status of clients. The goals for this chapter are to better prepare the fitness professional to deal one-on-one with new clients and to help them make their first sessions with new clients run as smoothly as possible. For more on this topic, visit Joe-Cannon.com and read the post entitled, *"Certified but never trained anyone: What to do."*

The Initial Interview

The initial interview is the first meeting that a fitness professional has with a new client. This time can be used to gather valuable information as well as to demonstrate to the new client one's proficiency and professionalism. The initial interview should be conducted in a private area such as an office or cubical, if possible. This is not only because the client may divulge sensitive information such as personal contact information, but also because it can help assuage uneasiness that the client might feel during any testing that occurs. Taking circumference or body fat measurements in a public area is one of the fastest ways to make a new client feel uneasy and to demonstrate a lack of professionalism. While this may not be an issue for fitness trainers who travel to people's homes, for health clubs that are space-limited, this can be a difficult obstacle to overcome. However, health clubs that wish to improve profit margins by incorporating premium services such as nutrition counseling or personal training should take steps to designate a private area specifically for this purpose.

The initial interview also gives the fitness professional and new client time to get to know each other and to engage in conversation. While on the surface, this may seem secondary to the main goals of the initial interview, this time together can aid in the gathering of valuable information. For example, consider body language. It has been said that only 20% of a spoken sentence is verbal, while the other 80% is non-verbal. Body language, which includes factors such as posture, eye contact, firmness of handshake, folding of arms, and other non-verbal cues, can help the fitness professional understand a client's personality and level of motivation. Sitting timidly in a chair, not making eye contact, or not removing coats when indoors may be signs that the person is depressed or feels incapable of doing anything to improve his or her circumstances. Maybe the individual has tried every diet on the market and has worked with a fitness professional in the past without seeing any progress. Perhaps the person views you as their last hope! Recognizing a person's subconscious non-verbal signals can be a remarkable asset, because it will help you to better put their fears and anxieties to rest and may enable you to form a bond as well.

Fitness professionals, whether working independently or in a health club setting, should also provide their personal contact information such as cell phone number and/or email address. Business cards made on any home computer can make this easy to do. Providing this information will help the client schedule sessions as well as facilitate easy cancellation of training sessions if an emergency arises. Phone numbers should have voice mail so that clients can leave a message. If communicating via email, it is in the fitness professional's best interest to provide their clients with a *professional*, easy-to-spell email address. This can be something as simple as "yourname@yahoo.com". Pornographic or otherwise suggestive email addresses are inappropriate and off-putting to new clients.

The initial interview is also a good starting place to begin collecting general and medical history information. Much of this information is easily obtained by having the new client complete a medical or health history questionnaire, one of which is provided for your convenience in the Appendix section at the end of this book. All health history forms should contain several sections, which will be described below.

Personal Contact Information

Information such as name, address, phone number, email address, emergency contact information, and the client's primary care physician are listed here. All personal and medical history data collected should be kept private. Fitness professionals should also refrain from discussing a client's personal or private information with other colleagues in a way that would allow for the client to be identified. In addition, the client's specific conditions should not be discussed in public settings like restaurants. Personal trainers should keep all of their clients' information in an organized, secure filing system such as a filing cabinet that has the ability to be locked. This is especially important if the records are being maintained in a hospital setting such as a hospital-based fitness center, which may be subject to specific privacy regulations.

Personal Medical History

This section provides information regarding the client's personal medical status. Questions to ask in this section include those regarding diseases, syndromes, surgeries, and injuries. Other possible questions include those pertaining to cholesterol levels, blood pressure, and cigarette-smoking habits. Whether or not the client is currently exercising should also be addressed in this section.

Prior to working with clients with serious medical issues like heart disease, diabetes, and cancer, the fitness professional should refer them to their primary care physician to obtain a written approval note. This serves not only as an extra measure of safety for the individual, but also may protect the fitness professional in the event of litigation. Obtaining a note from a qualified medical professional can also been seen as a marketing opportunity. It may be difficult to keep in touch with physicians because they are busy with patients, paperwork, and other tasks that make demands on their time. However, referring high-risk clients back to their physicians prior to training may help the fitness professional inform doctors about their health services. More importantly, doing so speaks volumes to medical professionals about the level of competency and care that a fitness professional provides for patients.

Conditions that Warrant a Physician's Permission Prior to Exercise

• Heart disease	• Chest pain at rest	• Emphysema
• High blood pressure	• Chest pain during exercise	• Pregnancy
• Kidney disorders	• Diabetes	• Cancer
• Prior heart attack	• HIV/AIDS	• Asthma
• Pacemaker	• Morbid Obesity	• Sedentary lifestyle
• Heart surgery	• Early death of parents	• Stroke

Family Medical History

Most medical history forms have a section that inquires about the health of immediate family members. This information may shed light on issues that the client may encounter in the future. For example, knowing that a client's parents suffered from osteoporosis may help the fitness professional better counsel the client on strategies for minimizing the risk of osteoporosis later in life. It can also be seen as another opportunity to identify high-risk individuals. Research finds that those whose mother, sister, or daughter died suddenly before the age of 65 or father, brother, or son unexpectedly passed away before the age of 55 may have an increased risk of early death from heart disease.[2]

Medications

Personal trainers are generally not physicians or pharmacists. While some very good books and websites do exist to educate personal trainers on medications, diseases, and other conditions, asking about medication usage is not to prompt the fitness professional to attempt to analyze the effects of medications. Rather, the goal should solely to identify high-risk individuals. Clients using medications for serious medical conditions like high blood pressure (hypertension), diabetes, heart disease, kidney disorders, cancer, and others should be referred back to their physician prior to beginning an exercise program. A release note from a physician should be obtained for the fitness professional's records as well.

Dietary Supplement Use

Dietary supplements are very popular among people, so it is likely that clients will be using them or have used them in the past. While some supplements may help reduce disease risk factors in theory, many supplements lack peer-reviewed clinical evidence. Knowledge of a client's dietary supplement usage may allow the fitness professional to better educate their clients on well balanced nutrition habits. An excellent resource on this topic is *Nutritional Supplements: What Works and Why*, available at www.Joe-Cannon.com. You can also read my science-based reviews at www.Supplement-Geek.com.

Fitness History

Given the correlation of exercise with weight loss and reduced disease risk, the fitness professional may want to inquire about this aspect of health as well. Knowledge of someone's exercise history and preferences can help the personal trainer design an effective exercise program that is enjoyable and that addresses the client's specific needs. For example, clients indicating that they play a particular sport or activity give the personal trainer the opportunity to incorporate movements that may strengthen muscles to help them play their sport safely and with excellence.

PAR-Q

PAR-Q stands for Physical Activity Readiness Questionnaire and is a one-page form that can help the personal trainer identify people (ages 15–69) who may not be ready to begin an exercise program. Essentially, the PAR-Q asks a series of simple questions. Answering "yes" to any question on the PAR-Q means that the person may have a significant medical issue and should be referred to their physician before exercise training begins. Questions usually asked on the PAR-Q include:[2]

1. Has your doctor ever said that you have a heart condition and that you should only do physical activity recommended by a doctor?
2. Do you feel pain in your chest when you do physical activity?
3. In the past month, have you had chest pain when you were not doing physical activity?
4. Do you lose your balance because of dizziness or do you ever lose consciousness?
5. Do you have a bone or joint problem that could be made worse by a change in your physical activity?
6. Is your doctor currently prescribing drugs (for example, water pills) for your blood pressure or heart condition?
7. Do you know of any other reason why you should not do physical activity?

The questions in the PAR-Q can be incorporated into a section of a standard health history questionnaire or may be included on a separate form altogether. The actual PAR-Q form can be viewed online by connecting to an Internet search engine like Google™ and typing in the phrase "PAR-Q and You." Some people reading these words may be the owners of health clubs. By having all new members complete the PAR-Q before joining, you can effectively screen for many high-risk individuals and provide an added layer of protection for those who wish to start an exercise program.

The Liability Waiver

Fitness professionals, whether working at a health club or self-employed, should have all new clients sign a standard liability waiver. The liability waiver can offer some legal protection in the event of litigation. Fitness professionals should have an attorney create the waiver. Clients should not only sign the waiver, but should also understand it. In addition, liability insurance is absolutely necessary for all fitness trainers.

The Client/Trainer Agreement

The client/trainer agreement (or "contract") is a form that outlines the responsibilities of the fitness professional as well as those of the client. It is here that the fitness professional may list information that he or she feels is necessary and important for the client to know. Items that could be listed here include dressing appropriately, procedures and timing for fitness testing, cancellation policy, and training package duration. Some trainers may also use the form as a motivational tool. In other words, some people may be more likely to continue with personal training and make progress toward their goals if they sign their name to a form. This form is not legally binding and may be used at the trainer's discretion.

Setting and Achieving Goals

Before walking through the door to their first meeting with a fitness professional, new clients will undoubtedly have many goals that they would like to accomplish. The fitness professional should make certain that these goals are realistic and attainable. For example, the goal of losing 30 pounds in one month is not realistic or healthy and is probably not attainable for most people. Large goals should be broken up into smaller, more manageable and realistic goals. Thus, the fitness professional and the client should work together to modify unrealistic goals in this way. Breaking large, lofty goals into smaller, more manageable chunks will help prevent the client from becoming discouraged over time.

Fitness professionals are also fitness educators. One way in which personal trainers can educate their clients is by teaching people the power of writing down their goals. Studies show that, when people write their goals down on paper, they are more likely to achieve those goals in the long run. Some health clubs actually have that new clients complete to help the trainer get an idea of what the person wants to accomplish. The problem with this, however, is that everybody will probably have very similar goals (e.g., to lose weight or to tone up), and the more the trainer sees the same thing over and over, the less likely he or she is to pay attention to it. That being said, there are other more effective ways to list goals.

When setting goals, clients should be encouraged to write their goals out, to be as specific as possible, and to give the reasons why they want to achieve those goals. The phrase "I want to lose weight" is vague and probably is not going to remain meaningful over time. A better written goal is, "I want to decrease my weight by 20 pounds because it will help reduce the pain I feel in my knees and help lower my blood pressure." Obviously, goals written like this require some thought on the part of the client, so assigning this task as "homework" may be necessary. This idea of "homework" can actually be a good thing because when clients sit down in private, they may really start to think about the real reasons why they want to achieve their goals. When doing this exercise, the client should be as honest and frank as possible and should hold nothing back. Reassure him or her that nobody will ever view what has been written. This is crucial because what they write will probably be their private, innermost thoughts and feelings. Having people commit to writing their goals in this way helps them take ownership of those goals. In essence, they have taken a small step. By committing to a small step like this, they are more likely to take the bigger step of achieving their goals!

Once the fitness professional has the client's goals and has broken them down into attainable short- and long-term objectives, he or she should review the goals on a regular basis with the client. This also should occur in private. Fitness professionals should sit down with the client and, with clipboard in hand, ask questions such as "What have you done over the past week to achieve your goals?" and "What have been your setbacks, if any?" All answers should be written down and techniques to address overcoming obstacles should be identified. Progress should also be praised to help spur the client toward the continuation of goal achievement. For more on working with clients, see my book, *Personal Fitness Training: Beyond the Basics*, available at Joe-Cannon.com.

Nutrition Assessment

Prior to giving specific nutrition advice, the fitness professional should have clients complete a personal nutrition assessment. A nutrition assessment is simply a written record of what foods a person has consumed over a specified time period. One of the most common methods is to have clients write down what they consumed over a 3-day period. This is sometimes called a *3-day food diary*. Information to report in the food diary can include:

- What food was consumed?
- Amount of food that was consumed?
- What time was the food was consumed?
- Was the person hungry when food was consumed?
- How were they feeling (e.g., happy, sad, etc.)?

This information will give valuable insights into not only the eating habits of clients, but also into what provokes them to eat. For example, it may be noticed that when a client is sad or depressed, he or she eats large amounts of high-calorie foods. This information may allow the client to take steps to avoid high-calorie foods during times of stress or depression. It is important that, while keeping a food diary, the client eats normally and does not substitute foods that he or she feels the fitness professional would want them to eat. It is also important that the days listed on the 3-day food record represent typical days. Days that are not typical, including special events such as weddings and others, should not be included in the 3-day food log.

Clients should strive to be as specific as possible about the types of foods they are eating. For example, listing "soda" is not as specific as listing "12 ounces of diet orange soda." "One slice of bread" is better reported as "one slice of whole-wheat bread." Being specific can be a double-edged sword, however, because people who become overly precise may begin actually measuring their food. This could lead to an underreporting of what is actually consumed. Similarly, people should not weigh the food that they eat because this also may lead to underreporting. An abbreviated sample of a food journal created with Microsoft Excel is shown here:

Sample 3-Day Food Diary

Time of Day	Place Food was Consumed	What was Consumed	Amount Eaten or Calories	Feelings
Day 1				
Day 2				
Day 3				

Obviously, the journal depicted above is a very simple example of what can be made on anyone's home computer. Another alternative to making a food journal yourself is to reach out to pharmaceutical representatives for assistance. Pharmaceutical representatives have a wide assortment of items that they routinely give to doctors and other health care professionals to help advertise their products. Keep in mind that these free journals will likely bear advertisements for a weight loss medication, something that fitness trainers may be opposed to. Another alternative is to use apps and websites that let people easily track their food (and exercise) from their cell phone or computer.

It is important to make it clear to clients that the purpose behind a food journal is not to make them feel guilty about what they are eating, but to help them gain insights into what they are eating. While writing down what was eaten is probably not something that a person should do forever, occasionally completing a food journal may provide the individual with feedback on their eating choices and may help keep them on track over time.

Obstacles to Progress

Many clients will undoubtedly encounter areas that hinder goal attainment. For example, some clients may find it difficult to abstain from purchasing high-calorie, high-fat foods when shopping at the supermarket. Clients may not be aware of the fact that supermarkets are designed in a way that keeps consumers in the stores for as long as possible. The longer they are in the store looking for something, the more items they encounter and the more they are tempted to buy (see the chapter "Supermarket Self-Defense"). To help combat this, the fitness professional may suggest that the client eat prior to shopping to nullify urges to purchase what is not needed. Going to the supermarket with a shopping list can also help keep people on track. By having a shopping list, people know exactly what they need and spend less time roaming around aimlessly. Personal trainers may also want to accompany clients to the supermarket or hold seminars for clients on how to read food labels.

Record Keeping

The fitness professional should maintain up-to-date records on all clients. This begins with the very first meeting and continues throughout the relationship with the client. Each meeting with the client should be documented and the record placed in the client's folder for easy retrieval if needed at a future date. Information that should be recorded at each meeting includes:

- The date of the meeting
- Issues discussed during the meeting
- Areas in which the client is having difficulty and areas in which he or she is excelling
- Areas for future follow-up (e.g., asking the client to present the 3-day food journal at your next meeting)

In addition, the fitness trainer should record other valuable information, such as the client's weight, percent body of fat, body circumferences, and BMI, at regular intervals. These measurements do not have to be taken at every meeting, but should be taken at intervals spaced far enough apart for a picture of the client's progress to be tracked over time. The client should not be made to feel uncomfortable during these measurements. Rather, personal trainers should reinforce the fact that these calculations are part of the "big picture," which is the ultimate improvement of the health of the individual. Along with these measurements, the professional should also record other improvements and obstacles to progress that the client may volunteer during routine conversations. Examples may include reductions in clothing size, reductions in cholesterol levels, or improvements in performing activities of daily living such as walking up stairs.

While some may choose to keep track of clients' data on a computer, it is also recommended that backup copies be made at regular intervals to minimize the loss of data which may occur during a computer mishap.

Body Composition Analysis

Fat can be divided into two different reserves: *essential fat* and *storage fat*. Essential fat represents the fat that is needed for the body to continue to carry out normal life processes. Essential fat consists of fat in the liver, spleen, bone marrow, muscles, intestines, and the central nervous system.[36] Essential fat represents only about 3% of total body fat in men and about 12% of fat in women.[36] Storage fat includes all fat reserves above and beyond essential fat. Average percentages of body fat are 12%–18% for college-age men and 16%–25% for college-age women.[27] Obesity is defined as body fat in excess of 25% for men and 30% for women.[27] Many studies find that disease risk increases as body fat increases. Research also notes that the location where fat is stored plays a role in disease development. For example, men tend to store much of their fat around their abdomen. This fat distribution pattern is linked to greater rates of heart disease than that seen in females, who tend to store much fat around the hips and thighs.

Body Fat Percentages		
	Men	**Women**
Average	12%–18%	16%–25%
Obese	> 25%	> 30%

Body composition refers to the relative amounts of fat and muscle in the body. While many individuals use a household scale to estimate their weight, a scale usually only provides one raw number, total body weight, which does not distinguish between muscle and fat. While the scale can help keep people on track, other tools are also available that can provide deeper insights into a person's body composition. Some methods are, of course, better than others, and all have their drawbacks. The fitness professional should have an understanding of the different methods available to assess body composition in order to help his or her clients reach their maximum potential while reducing the incidence of a variety of diseases. To help with this, the following overview of various popular body composition analysis techniques is offered.

Body Typing

This is an older method that attempts to classify people into one of three types: *ectomorph*, *mesomorph,* and *endomorph*. The ectomorph is said to be thin and have a difficult time gaining weight. Endomorphs are said to be at the other end of the spectrum, as they are round and have a difficult time losing weight. Mesomorphs are said to have a muscular build and narrow waist. Problems with this type of analysis include the fact that it does not consider percentage of body fat and not everybody fits into these classifications—some may be composites of each. Also, classifying people as specific body types may provide people with a "crutch" that prevents them from attaining their goals.

Height–Weight Tables

Height-weight tables assess body composition based on gender and the size of one's frame. Like scales, height-weight tables do not assess the amount of body fat a person has. Rather, they compare people to the "average" person. Problems abound when using these tables for body composition analysis. For example, many professional athletes are considered overweight when assessed using height-weight tables.[36] Due to error and because better alternative methods exist, the fitness professional should not rely solely on height-weight tables to determine body composition.

Body Mass Index

The body mass index (BMI) is calculated using this equation:

$$\text{Weight (in kilograms)} \div \text{height (in meters}^2)$$

That is, one calculates BMI as the weight of a person (in kilograms) divided by the person's height (in meters squared). This is written in the form "kg/m^2." For example, if a person weighs 200 pounds and is 6 feet tall, his BMI is calculated in the following way:

1. Convert pounds to kilograms. Since there are 2.2 pounds in a kilogram, 200 pounds ÷ 2.2 = 90 kilograms.

2. Convert the person's height to meters squared (m^2). Since the person is 6 feet tall and since there are 3 feet in a meter, the person is 2 meters tall. Then, square this amount (that multiply 2 meters x 2 meters) to get 4 m^2.

3. The person's BMI is 90 kg ÷ 4 m^2 = $\boxed{22.5 \text{ kg/m}^2}$

BMI is sometimes useful as a quick assessment of a person's risk of disease because obesity-related health problems increase as BMI increases over 25 kg/m^2 for most people.[2] According to current guidelines, a BMI of 25–29 kg/m^2 is classified as "overweight" and a BMI of over 30 kg/m^2 is considered "obese." A BMI of 40 or more is classified as "extremely high," which is associated with a very high risk of obesity-related diseases.[2] While BMI offers a quick and relatively easy way to assess a person's body composition, it does have its limitations. For example, like the height-weight tables described previously, many athletes (who have a low body fat percentage) would be classified as "obese" according to the BMI determination. Looking at this from another point of view, BMI does not differentiate between muscle and fat. Two people can be the same height and weight and thus have the same BMI, yet one person may have a body fat percentage of 10% while another may be 35%. In addition, there is a ±5% error when determining body fatness from BMI.[2] Thus, caution should be used when labeling a person "overweight" or "obese" from the calculation of BMI alone.

Body Mass Index Values	
BMI (kg/m2)	Meaning
Less than 18.5	Underweight
18.5 - 24.9	Normal weight
25.0 -29.9	Overweight
Greater than 30	Obese

Circumference Measurements

The advantage of circumference measurements is that they are quick and easy and only require a tape measure that the fitness professional uses to measure the circumferences of various body areas. This information can be plugged into equations to estimate body composition or can be used to track changes over time. Alternatively, the measurements themselves can be used by themselves as a check of progress. The major disadvantage of this type of body composition analysis is that it gives little information about the amounts of fat and muscle that a person has. Nevertheless, for the fitness professional working with morbidly obese individuals, this method offers a way to track changes while at the same time not making the client feel overly self-conscious. The following table lists areas that are commonly measured for girth.

Circumference Measurements

Area	Where Measurement is Taken
Neck	Distance around the neck
Waist	Most narrow part of the torso
Abdomen	At the umbilicus (belly button)
Hips	Maximal circumference of the buttocks
Thighs	Largest circumference of the thigh
Calf	Maximal circumference of the calf
Chest	Around mid-sternum, just above the nipple line
Upper arm	Around the midpoint of the upper arm
Forearm	Maximum girth of the forearm

When measuring limb circumferences, do so in the straightened, unflexed position. This will provide information on the limb's resting circumference. While some may choose to measure only the right limbs, both sides can be measured if desired. Fitness professionals working with very obese people should keep in mind that they may be unable to measure abdominal circumference because of excess abnormal fat. Those wanting to avoid possible embarrassing situations may wish to not measure this area in morbidly obese individuals.

From circumference measurements, it is possible to calculate the *waist to hip ratio* (sometimes abbreviated *"WHR"*). The waist to hip ratio is often used to estimate the degree of abdominal obesity, which is seen as a greater risk for heart disease than fat relegated to the hip and thigh areas. In other words, as WHR increases, the risk of obesity-related diseases also increases.[2] A waist to hip ratio of greater than 0.95 for adult men or 0.86 for adult women indicates that individuals are at greater risk of developing diseases associated with being overweight.[28]

It is important to remember that professional athletes may have a very high WHR when they are actually at low risk for obesity-related diseases. Thus, the WHR should be used as a general guideline, not as the definitive measure of obesity. In other words, it is possible to have a high WHR and not be obese at all.

Alternately, waist circumference alone can be used to estimate disease risk. Men with a circumference greater than 40 inches and women with a circumference greater than 35 inches are said to be have an increased risk of obesity-related diseases. In fact, research suggests that waist circumference alone is a better predictor than BMI.[131]

Skin Fold Analysis

Another way to estimate body composition is by using special calipers that essentially pinch people at different parts of the body to measure fat beneath the skin. This method is possible because a relationship exists between the fat just under the skin and one's total amount of body fat.[27] The caliper device measures the thickness of various skin folds, then this information is plugged into equations to calculate an estimation of body composition. When performed correctly, the skin fold technique may be accurate to about ± 3%. Various equations exist for skinfold analysis of body composition, with each using different sites to be pinched. When using skin fold analysis, make sure that the equation you are using corresponds to the sites you are pinching. For example, there is an equation specific to testing only three sites. Fitness professionals must make sure that they measure the sites specified by a given equation, as measuring the wrong sites reduces accuracy. Also, skin fold measurements are always taken on the right side of the body only. While research shows that skin fold analysis can provide relatively good estimates of body composition when done properly, some drawbacks to this technique include the following:

1. Total body fat does not just depend on the fat under the skin. Skin fold analysis cannot measure fat around organs.

2. The degree of accuracy of skin fold analysis depends on the expertise of the person performing the test.

3. Equations for this method are gender-, age-, and race-specific. Thus, using the wrong equation will generate a less accurate result.

4. Some people are not comfortable being pinched by people whom they do not know.

5. This method may not be appropriate for the very obese.

Bioelectric Impedance Analysis

Bioelectric impedance analysis (BIA) represents an easy-to-administer technique for assessing body composition, which makes it very popular in fitness and wellness centers. Bioelectric impedance analysis works by passing a low intensity electric current through the body and measuring its resistance.[2] Because fat is not a good conductor of electricity, the greater the fat mass a person has, the greater the resistance and the slower the current passes through the body. In this way, BIA is able to provide a quick and relatively accurate estimate of body composition. BIA devices usually cost about $50 and come in hand-held versions and other versions upon which a person can stand. In addition to estimating percent body fat, some models may calculate BMI as well. Some models may have an "athlete mode" that provides a greater degree of accuracy for those who exercise on a regular basis. Whichever type is chosen, the accuracy of BIA depends on several guidelines, which are outlined here.

General BIA Guidelines

1. Do not eat or drink for at least four hours before the test.
2. Do not exercise for at least 12 hours before the test.
3. Do urinate 30 minutes before the test.
4. Do not drink alcohol for at least 48 hours before the test.
5. Do not ingest any diuretics (including caffeine) before the test unless prescribed by a physician to do so.

Another factor to consider with BIA is the equation being used to determine body composition.[2] Many BIA equations exist. The equations used today in commercially available machines are probably good for most individuals, but some machines may be unable to determine body composition for those falling outside of the scope of what the machine "thinks" is normal. People for whom the machine may be unable to determine body compassion include those over 300 pounds as well as bodybuilders and other professional athletes who have unusually low body fat percentages.

One group in whom BIA should not be used includes those who have pacemakers, defibrillators, or other implantable heart devices, as the electrical signal may accidentally activate these machines. Fitness professionals should ask everyone, regardless of age, about whether they have a pacemaker, defibrillator, or similar device. Likewise, BIA should not be performed on pregnant women.

Near Infrared Interactance

The estimation of body composition by near infrared interactance (NIR) makes use of a specialized probe that is placed against an area of the body (e.g., the biceps) and emits infrared light that is passed through muscle and fat. Fat and muscle will absorb different frequencies of light. The difference between them is entered into prediction equations along with information on age, height, weight, and activity level to estimate body composition. While variations of this technique have been used in clinical settings since the 1960s, portable devices that are commercially available have been shown to be less accurate than the skin fold techniques and bioelectric impedance analysis described above. Some research hints that NIR may be less accurate in those who exercise.[123] Other research finds that NIR might overestimate body fatness in lean people and underestimate it in overweight people. More study is needed before NIR is universally accepted.

Hydrostatic Weighing

Hydrostatic weighing is often called the "gold standard" of body composition analysis because it is the most accurate method and the basis upon which all the others are compared. Because of this, hydrostatic weighing is often used in clinical research. The other name for this technique is "underwater weighing," a phrase derived from the fact that individuals are completely submerged in water to determine body composition. Hydrostatic weighing is based on *Archimedes's Principle*—that is, a body buoyed in water will be forced to the surface by a force equal to the volume of water that it displaces. Stating this another way, fat floats, and the more fat a person has on his or her body, the lighter the person will be when weighed under the water. When having body composition determined by this method, the person usually sits on a specialized scale and is completely submerged in water. The individual then forcibly exhales as much air out of his or her lungs as possible and remains motionless. For individuals who are uncomfortable with being submerged under the water as well as for those who are not comfortable being in a bathing suit, this method can be a frightening experience. Because special equipment is required, underwater weighing is more likely to be offered at a university that has a physical education department as opposed to a health club setting.

Air Displacement

Just as hydrostatic weighing measures the displacement of water, body composition can also be determined by measuring the amount of air that a person displaces. The most popular of these types of machines is the Bod Pod®, which measures air displacement when people sit in a special chamber. Clinical studies have been published on the Bod Pod, and some find it to be almost as accurate as hydrostatic weighing in a variety of populations.[34, 53] While body composition can be determined in a matter of minutes, one possible drawback is the price, which can be tens of thousands of dollars. In addition, not all studies have found air displacement to be as accurate as hydrostatic weighing for all individuals.[33, 55, 56] Thus, more research is warranted on air displacement before it is universally accepted for all populations.

Dual Energy X-Ray Absorptiometry

In addition to its more common use (determining bone density) dual energy x-ray absorptiometry (also called "DEXA Scan") can also very precisely estimate the amount of fat and lean muscle tissue present in one's body. Like the Bod Pod® described above, DEXA is quite expensive. More importantly, because it uses low-level radiation, DEXA is very unlikely to be found at any health club but is reserved for hospitals and other clinical research settings.

Chapter 11

Diets and Weight Loss

Americans spend over 30 billion dollars a year on a myriad of books, potions, pills, and exercise devices touted to aid in shedding excess bodyweight.[38] The reality, however, is that 95% of any weight that is lost by these methods is probably regained eventually. Another sad reality is that the vast majority of diets do not appear to work long-term for all people. This makes the job of the fitness professional, who espouses the time-tested concepts of "calories in" and "calories out," to be especially difficult. In reality, however, this is actually the premise of many popular diets spoken of by people today. In other words, most diets encourage people to reduce the number of calories that they eat. This chapter will deal with many of the most popular diets on the market today. The goal for this chapter is to arm the fitness professional with the knowledge needed to help their clients safely navigate though the hype and through the odd approaches that seem to be all-too-common in the world of weight loss.

Low-Carb Diets

By far, one of the most popular diets in recent history has been the low-carbohydrate diet. Low-carb diets are sometimes called ketogenic diets because they tend to produce acid-like molecules called ketones.

People usually report losing a significant amount of weight during the first few weeks of a low-carbohydrate diet. There is actually a very good reason for this. All humans store excess carbohydrates in the form of glycogen. When carbohydrates are not eaten or when their intake is severely curtailed, the body slowly starts to break down its stored glycogen reserves to maintain blood sugar levels. As glycogen is degraded to glucose, a lot of water is also released in the process. In fact, every gram of glycogen liberates about 3 grams of water. This is why one of the first things that people notice while on a low-carb diet is the almost constant urge to urinate. After a week or two, a significant amount of weight is lost, but most of it is in the form of water. Low-carb diets can be rather difficult to maintain over time because carbohydrates are our body's preferred fuel source. This lack of carbs can lead to fatigue and a decrease in aerobic exercise capacity. While the long-term safety of low-carb diets in terms of cardiovascular health is still not known, studies to date generally find them safe for short-term usage. Research, however, hints that long-term use may not be more effective than simply eating less. In one of the longest studies of this diet to date, 63 overweight individuals were followed for one year.[124] About half of the individuals followed the Atkins diet, while the other half ate a lower-calorie diet (1,200-1,800 calories per day), with the majority of calories (60%) coming from carbohydrates. For the first 6 months, the Atkins group lost about 4% more weight than the calorie counting group. However, after one year, there was no significant difference in the amount of weight lost by either group. A longer study was published in the *New England Journal of Medicine* in 2008.[132] This study lasted two years and found that an Atkins-type diet (where 40% of calories came from fat) resulted in more weight loss than a low-fat or Mediterranean-type diet that used 30% and 33% fat, respectively. The average weight loss for the low-carb group was 10.3 pounds over the two-year course of the study. The low-fat and Mediterranean groups lost 6.3 and 9.7 pounds, respectively. Thus, the difference in weight lost between the groups was not significant. In addition, considering the two-year duration of the study, relatively little weight was lost across the board. All groups were highly monitored by researchers, and the low-carb group was advised to keep their intake of saturated and trans fats low. This, either alone or in combination with the weight loss, may have resulted in the favorable effects on the cholesterol/HDL ratio noticed in the low-carb group. For more information, see the post located at www.joe-cannon.com/low-carb-diets-how-they-work/.

High-Protein Diets

High-protein diets require individuals to consume large amounts of dietary protein, often in excess of the RDA (0.8 g/kg BW). Proponents of high-protein diets claim that elevated protein intakes may lead to weight loss because protein may temporarily suppress the appetite and force the body to rely on fat as a fuel source.[36] A more logical reason, however, is related to water loss associated with glycogen depletion. Very high-protein diets (several times the RDA) may also be accompanied by unwanted side effects such as electrolyte imbalances and altered pH levels via ketone accumulation.[45] On the plus side, kidney problems resulting from high-protein diets appear to be less of an issue than once thought.[72] Protein does tend to slow digestion and also seems to raise metabolism more than carbohydrate or fat. Another mechanism that may be responsible for the weight loss observed on these diets is that protein does not contain a lot of calories (only 4 calories per gram). While a slightly higher level of protein may help some people reduce weight, a problem arises when protein is consumed at the expense of other healthy foods that the body also needs. People who advocate high-protein diets usually forget that all food may be "health food" when used in moderation. High intakes of protein are not advised for people with kidney or liver disease because it may make their condition worse.

Low-Fat Diets

Before low-carbohydrate diets, there were low-fat diets. At the heart of many low-fat diets is a reduction in calories. Thus, many low-fat diets are also low-calorie diets. Each gram of fat has 9 calories—more than either protein or carbohydrate (each has about 4 calories per gram). When people begin cutting fat out of their diet (or reducing fat grams), they are really cutting back on a lot of calories. These types of diets also tend to place an emphasis on fruits and vegetables, which are also low in calories. From a health perspective, a low-fat, high-fruit and vegetable diet may be beneficial because high-fat diets have been linked to diseases such as some cancers and heart disease.

Low-fat diets that also emphasize fruits and vegetables may be effective because of the phytonutrient content of these foods, and emerging evidence suggests that consuming fresh produce may also reduce disease risk. However, the bottom line is this: from a health standpoint, low-fat diets may have advantages, but from a weight loss standpoint, most are just low in calories.

Of all low-fat diets, one in particular stands out. It is called the *Ornish Diet* and was named after Dean Ornish, a medical doctor and researcher. The Ornish diet consists of a very low-fat diet (about 10% of total calories coming from fat), daily aerobic exercise, and stress reduction techniques like meditation. Research on the Ornish diet has noted that it can help weight loss.[125] However, another reason why some may be interested in the Ornish Diet has to do findings that it can lead to significant reductions in plaque buildup after sticking with the diet for up to a year. Research notes that the Ornish Diet may lower LDL (bad cholesterol) as well as C-reactive protein (CRP), which are implicated in heart disease development. The Ornish Diet also places an emphasis on daily, moderate intensity aerobic exercise to help boost HDL and burn calories. Because stress can also contribute to heart disease, another aspect of the Ornish plan is its emphasis on stress reduction techniques like yoga, mediation, and social support.

Acid/Alkaline Diets

"Alkaline good, acid bad." This premise suggests that when our bodies become too "acid" by eating the wrong foods, weight gain and disease develop. Foods said to make us more "acid" include meat, poultry, milk, and grains. Caffeine and alcohol are also usually off-limits. Foods that are more "alkaline" include fruits and vegetables. Thus, alkaline-based diets tend to contain a lot of healthy, low-calorie foods.

When delving into these types of diets, readers quickly encounter the term *pH*, so let us define it here. The pH refers to the degree of acidity, which is related to the number of hydrogen atoms present (this is the source for the "H" in "pH"). The pH scale is from 0–14, where a rating of 0 is very acid and a pH of 14 is very alkaline (also called basic). Different parts of the body range in their degree of acidity or alkalinity. For example, human blood has a normal pH of about 7.35–7.4 (alkaline), while the stomach has a pH of about 1–3 (acid). It is important to remember that the body wants to maintain its "normal" pH—and for good reason. For example, if the blood could not maintain its normal (alkaline) state, a glass of orange juice might kill us! As such, it's debatable if alkaline-type diets can significantly alter body pH for any length of time.

There have been preliminary studies on alkaline diets, but some of them appear to have methodological problems.[143] For example, some studies used alkalizing supplements (like sodium bicarbonate) rather than foods to demonstrate effects. On the plus side, diets that are said to make us more "alkaline" tend to contain fruits and vegetables, which are healthy. As such, it seems more plausible that any weight loss seen with these diets might be more associated with increased fruit and vegetable consumption coupled with eating fewer calories than with "becoming more alkaline."

Sometimes people on these diets are instructed to measure pH by testing their saliva or urine. One problem with doing this is that saliva and urine pH may not be the same as the pH inside the body. As a result, testing these fluids may not be reliable indicators.

Cabbage Soup Diet

The cabbage soup diet has been around for decades, and many people still believe that there is something magical about this method. However, in reality, nothing can be further from the truth. How many calories are in cabbage soup? Not many. By eating only cabbage soup or mostly cabbage soup, people eliminate a large number of calories, which signals the body to begin breaking down its glycogen reserves. As mentioned previously, this releases a large volume of water into the circulatory system, resulting in frequent trips to the bathroom. Thus, while the cabbage soup diet might promote short-term water weight loss, in the long run, it is difficult to maintain because it is boring and humans need more than cabbage soup to survive and thrive. The cabbage soup diet is an example of many one-food-centered diets that abound on the internet. Another classic variation is the grapefruit diet. It, too, is a simply a low-calorie diet.

Blood Type-Based Diets

Blood type-based diets advocate that a person's blood type determines what foods can be eaten. Eating "right for your blood type," say advocates, can help reduce weight as well as improve overall health. For example, a person with type A blood might avoid meats and predominately eat vegetables. A person with type O blood should eat a high-protein, low-carbohydrate diet. The problem with blood type diets is that they have not been rigorously tested to see whether there is something to them. At least one study has noted that blood type plays no role in weight loss.[144]

Food Combining Diets

Some diet books are based on the notion that humans cannot adequately digest and absorb certain combinations of foods when they are eaten in the same meal. For example, some variations may state that carbohydrates should not be eaten with meats or that people should not eat fruit and meat in the same meal. According to these diets, weight loss and health results when the "correct" combinations of foods are eaten. Unfortunately, the bulk of the published, peer-reviewed nutrition and medical literature does not support the theory that we can only absorb certain combinations of foods or that only certain groupings of foods promote weight loss. Some variations of this diet regimen call for eating only fruits or only vegetables for the first week or two. Because fruits and vegetables tend to be low in calories, this might be the reason why people lose weight with this type of diet.

Zone-Type Diets

Some diets advocate that weight loss can only occur when people eat carbohydrates, proteins, and fats in specific percentages. While several variations of this concept exist, the most popular over the last decade has been the *Zone Diet* which advocates that weight loss and improved health are found by striving to have each meal be composed of 40% carbohydrate, 30% protein, and 30% fat. It is said that eating foods in these specific combinations puts one in the "zone." At the heart of many of these diets is the claim that eating foods in the 40-30-30 ratio will stabilize insulin levels. According to advocates, insulin, while a vital hormone, is responsible for obesity and various diseases. While the carbohydrate amount specified in these diets (40%) is less than that advocated by many nutrition educators, these diets are overall pretty healthy. Most diets emphasize fruits, vegetables, lean meats, and low fat products and restrict indulgence in foods containing saturated fats. Some have criticized these diets because they tend to be relatively low in calcium and whole grains.[127] One drawback to Zone-type diets is that it may be difficult to precisely calculate the proportions specified. However, because they do not totally eliminate any one food group, people may find it easier to stick with them over time. The fact that the Zone Diet emphasizes fruits and vegetables at every meal probably means that it is low in calories. Some research has been conducted on the Zone Diet and has found that it can help reduce weight.[125] Whether this effect is due to the diet decreasing insulin levels or because it is a low-calorie diet requires further research.

Raw Food Diets

Advocates of raw food diets feel that most, if not all, cooked foods are bad for us and that health and weight loss are best achieved when eating food in its natural state (raw). According to the raw food diet theory, by not cooking foods, one preserves enzymes and other vital nutrients that help keep us healthy. Raw food-based diets tend to be filled with nutrient-dense fruits and vegetables and low in calories. This reduction in calorie content is probably the reason why these diets reduce weight. Raw food diets also tend to emphasize organically grown foods, which contain far fewer chemicals, hormones, pesticides, and antibiotics. These diets are also usually low in fat (especially saturated fat) and have a higher fiber content, which helps slow digestion, making people feel fuller longer. On the other hand, some nutrients like lycopene and beta carotene, for example, are more bioavailable after cooking. In theory, some variations of raw food diets may be deficient in nutrients like vitamin B_{12} and calcium. Eating foods in their raw state may make it difficult for some with digestion problems as well. Overall, diets based on raw foods are pretty healthy and most likely will result in weight loss because of their emphasis on nutrient-dense, low-calorie fruits and vegetables. Diets of this type might also reduce the risk of several diseases like cancer, diabetes, and heart disease. Depending on how "back to the basics" a person gets with raw food diets, a good multivitamin as well as a calcium supplement might be something to consider.

Body For Life®

The Body For Life® program was developed by the makers of the EAS line of dietary supplements and popularized by the book *Body For Life* by Bill Philips. One of the advantages of this program is that it is less of a diet than a lifestyle change plan. The program emphasizes eating about 6 meals per day with each meal consisting of about 300 calories (about 1,800 calories per day are eaten). This is less than many people already eat, so this program is likely to promote weight loss. Each meal on this plan should also contain some lean protein like chicken or fish to help raise metabolism and promote muscle growth.

In addition, the Body For Life program does something that most other diets do not do—it places a heavy emphasis on exercise, specifically strength training. In a nutshell, the program advocates a pyramid-up system of strength training whereby a person lifts a weight for 12 reps, followed by a set of 10 reps, followed by a set of 8 reps, and finishes with a set of 6 reps. Rest periods of approximately 30 seconds–1 minute are taken between sets. Cardiovascular exercise is limited to about 20 minutes at a high intensity. Needless to say, this is a very aggressive strength training program, and beginners might want to do at least a month of strength training at lower intensities to prepare for it. One of the most interesting aspects of Body For Life is its emphasis on making smart food choices and trying to encourage people to determine why they make bad choices. This might make this program more well-rounded than other diets.

Diet Program	Emphasis	How it Works / Notes
Atkins Diet	Reduce carbohydrates.	Glycogen/water loss in beginning. Possible consumption of fewer calories long-term.
High-Protein Diets	Higher protein intakes.	Glycogen/water loss in beginning. Protein may boost metabolism and slow digestion.
Low Fat Diets	Reduce fat consumption.	Reducing fat really reduces calories. Low fat diets may reduce disease risk.
Acid/Alkaline Diets	Eat more alkaline foods like fruits and vegetables.	Fruits and vegetables are low in calories. Diet's impact on disease reduction is unknown.
Cabbage Soup diet	Eat cabbage soup.	Cabbage soup is low in calories. Promotes glycogen and water loss.

Diet Program	Emphasis	How it Works / Notes
Grapefruit Diet	Eat grapefruit.	Grapefruit is low in calories. Promotes glycogen and water loss. Grapefruit not appropriate for people using some medications
Blood Type-Based Diets	Eat foods according to your blood type.	No published peer-reviewed evidence to support diet's claims.
Food Combining Diets	Eat only specific combinations of foods.	No published peer-reviewed evidence to support diet's claims.
Zone-Type Diets	Eat Fruits, vegetables, lean meats in 40%–30%–30% combination.	Diet is low in calories.
Raw Food Diets	Eat only or mostly foods in their raw state.	Diet is low in calories.
Body For Life Diet	Eat several small means during the day plus regular exercise.	Low-calories plus exercise promotes weight loss/gain in muscle.
Ornish Diet	Eat a very low-fat diet plus daily aerobic exercise & stress reduction.	Diet is low in calories. Only diet to date clinically shown to reverse artery clogging plaque.

Questions to Ask about Diets

The following is a series of questions to ask when researching a diet:

1. How is the diet different from all others on the market?
2. Is the diet a low-calorie diet?
3. Is there any published research on the diet that proves it works?
4. Does the diet recommend or advocate questionable dietary supplements to help "support" weight loss? If yes, ask for published peer-reviewed research that proves the products work. See Supplement-Geek.com for more insights.
5. Does the diet program advocate restricting any single food group? If yes, this is probably unhealthy.
6. Is the diet something people can easily fit into their lifestyle for the long run?

Fitness professionals should remember that most diets will probably work in the short term. However, the fact that the majority of diets fail means that most have a miserable long-term track record. Diets are a short-term fix and nothing more. One of the toughest challenges facing fitness professionals today is helping people realize that real change comes not with the latest fad diet, but from recognizing the lifestyle habits that brought them to where they are now and taking reasonable and attainable steps toward a healthier way of life.

Chapter 12

Supermarket Self-Defense

Health and fitness guru Jack LaLanne once remarked, "Dying is easy. Staying alive is the hard part." Jack was right. Staying healthy is a 24/7 job to be sure. For some, working out may be the easy part because it requires a tangible effort. The more difficult area for people may be eating well, and for many, there is no greater temptation to overindulge than their local supermarket. This makes perfect sense. Think about it—everything is right there at your fingertips, just waiting to be seen and eaten! Believe it or not, supermarkets are actually designed this way on purpose. Everything in the supermarket is specifically arranged so that you will spend the maximum amount of time shopping. The longer you stay in the supermarket, the more money you will probably spend. Because there is a method to this madness, let us go over some of the design tactics used by today's big supermarket chains—as well as the local "mom-and-pop" stores in your neighborhood—to see how they encourage you to buy things that you might not ordinarily buy.

Did you ever notice that, whenever you enter a supermarket, you almost always have to walk through the fruit and vegetable section before you can get to the stuff you want? It is no accident that this is the case. Supermarket owners know (because they hire experts who do research on this) that the arrangement and aroma of all of those fruits and vegetables has a significant effect on people in terms of what they buy. An interesting fact about the produce section of supermarkets is that it may generate almost 20% of the supermarket's profits while only taking up about 10% of the store's space! The produce section is usually the second most profitable area in the typical supermarket. It is also not an accident that the veggies are found along the walls of most supermarkets. This is because a sizable amount of profit for the supermarket is generated by products lining the walls. Thus, the more time you spend hunting along the perimeter of the supermarket, the more money you are likely to spend.

If the produce section is the second most lucrative section in the supermarket, what do you think is the #1-ticket area? It is the meat section. Everybody (except maybe vegetarians) eats meat at least once in a while, so it makes perfect sense that this would be the area in which supermarkets generate the most revenue. The meat section is also strategically placed—usually along the back wall of the supermarket. The meat section is placed here so that you are more likely to run into it whenever you exit an isle. People, being the "Pavlovian dogs" that they are, say to themselves, "You know, I would really like to have hot dogs for dinner tonight!"

What about the dairy section? It is usually placed as far from the entrance as possible. The reason for this is that everybody usually buys milk or eggs when they go food shopping. Therefore, it is in the supermarket's best interest to lead you through as much of its gauntlet of goodies as possible before you arrive at the dairy section. In addition, when you finally arrive at the dairy section, you will find that popular items like milk are usually placed at one end of the dairy display, while stuff like butter is usually at the other end. This way, the supermarket gets you to look at all of the other less popular products in between.

Another way that supermarkets try to get you to buy goods is with the width of shopping carts. Sometimes the carts are so wide that it is hard to move through the narrow aisles of the supermarket. This is especially true if there are other shoppers in the aisle with you. The slower you move, the more likely you are to see something and buy it. Some have estimated that, for every unplanned extra minute we spend in the supermarket, we spend an extra $2.

What about those free samples that we are sometimes offered while shopping? Are they really free? Not really, especially if you decide to by the product. Free samples are another way that supermarkets entice us to buy what we ordinarily would not.

When you are in the checkout line, you are basically a captive audience with no place to go. While you are standing there waiting patiently, marketers hit you again with products that you might not ordinarily buy. Take a close look at those areas the next time you are at the market. What you will usually find is an assortment of candy, magazines, batteries, and even little toys. The toys and candy are strategically placed low to the ground, where small children can see them. Because adults are more likely to think about their breath, breath mints and similar items are placed higher up, closer to adult eye level. Some supermarkets even have TV displays that advertise products while you are waiting in line.

What about those "preferred customer cards" that supermarkets give out these days? While these cards do offer some discounts to those who present them at checkout, they are really designed to track the items that you buy so that the store can send you coupons encouraging you to buy more stuff.

The best way for people to protect themselves is to create a shopping list before going to the supermarket. Knowing ahead of time what you are going to buy will go a long way toward reducing the amount of time that you spend wandering aimlessly past the thousands of items clamoring for your attention.

Another way to protect yourself from buying items that you ordinarily would not purchase is to never go to the supermarket on an empty stomach. We are much more susceptible to the enticements of cookies, cakes, and other edible goodies when we arrive at the supermarket hungry.

The Big Picture

Deceptive as all of this may seem, in reality, it is really just capitalism, and supermarkets are not the only ones who do this. Supermarkets sell food just the same way as vitamin stores sell vitamins, car dealerships sell cars, health clubs sell fitness, and personal trainers sell health, fitness, knowledge, and hope. The goal of this chapter has not been to make you believe that there is a vast conspiracy to get people to eat, but rather to alert fitness professionals to these facts so that they can better equip people to make wise food choices. Some fitness professionals may want to go to the supermarket with their clients to help educate them further. For those who do this on a regular basis, it is probably wise to contact the supermarket ahead of time to make sure its ok. Some supermarkets catering to health-conscious people may even welcome the addition of a certified fitness professional and use him or her as a selling point. The bottom line is that, in moderation, all food is basically "health food." Helping people recognize this fact while avoiding the pitfalls of too much overindulgence is a laudable service that all fitness professionals should practice with their clients.

Jack LaLanne was mentioned at the start of this chapter. If you do not know who he was, See my blog post "Jack Lalanne The Biggest Name In Fitness History" to read just some of the ways that Jack changed the fitness world forever.

Chapter 13

Exercise & Weight Control

Exercise is an integral component of any sound weight loss program. Exercise burns calories and, along with reduced calorie intake, is one of the best tools that people can use to promote weight loss. Studies of the National Weight Control Registry, a database of people who were successful at long-term (i.e., longer than one year) weight loss, show that exercise was an important component of weight loss success. While many opt for aerobic exercise training when losing weight, resistance strength training can also help. Some even estimate that every pound of extra muscle can burn an extra 30–50 calories per day.[41] Thus, in theory, the greater the amount of lean muscle tissue one has, the greater the amount of overall calories one burns in a given time period. This, in turn, may lead to greater weight loss in the long run. In addition, evidence suggests that combining exercise with a reduced calorie intake enhances the amount of weight that is lost as fat.[9] Individuals most successful at losing weight and preventing the regaining of weight often report exercising at least 280 minutes per week.[1] This amounts to:

- 40 minutes per day if working out 7 days a week
- 56 minutes per day if working out 5 days a week
- 70 minutes per day if working out 4 days a week
- 93 minutes per day if working out 3 days a week

Notice that the numbers above are greater than the often quoted 30 minutes per day, 3–5 days per week for general cardiovascular health. Because not everybody can commit to large amounts of exercise on a daily basis, it is important to combine exercise with mild calorie restriction. Exercise alone is unlikely to cause significant weight loss in most people.

Types of Exercise

When deciding on an exercise program, people basically have two broad categories from which to choose: aerobic exercise (cardiovascular training) and anaerobic exercise (strength training). Both types of exercise offer advantages for the person looking to improve health, quality of life, and weight loss. As a general rule, aerobic exercise tends to burn a lot of calories during the activity. If opting for aerobic exercise, individuals should chose activities that incorporate the large muscles of the body such as the legs, chest, and back. Such exercises have a higher metabolic cost associated with them (i.e., they burn more calories). Health club machines that are appropriate for this include treadmills, steppers, elliptical machines, and rowers. For those not used to a regular exercise program, performing the activity 2–3 days a week and building up to 4–5 days a week is usually advocated. When designing an exercise program for a beginner, fitness professionals should place a greater emphasis on the duration of exercise rather than intensity of exercise. This is because greater exercise intensity is associated with greater risk of injury.

At the other end of the exercise spectrum is anaerobic exercise, which includes strength training. Strength training, while generally burning fewer calories than aerobic exercise, improves muscle strength and may elevate metabolic rate for some period of time after the activity ceases. Thus, strength training may help people burn more calories when they are sleeping! As with aerobic exercise, the emphasis here should also be on the large muscle groups of the body to maximize calorie utilization. People will burn more calories doing a chest press than when performing biceps curls, for example. Because many overweight individuals may not be accustomed to exercise, starting with one set of 10–15 repetitions for the major muscle groups of the body (e.g., chest, back, legs) will be easier and less likely to result in delayed onset muscle soreness (DOMS), a possible hindrance to the continuation of exercise. Generally, strength training should be performed 2–3 days a week.

When dealing with beginners, fitness professionals should be aware that exercise dropout rates increase when workouts last longer than 60 minutes. Because of this, circuit training might be ideal for new exercisers and for those trying to lose weight, because it offers a variety of exercises in a short period of time, is not perceived as boring, and places less stress on muscles and joints. Many fitness professionals are enthusiastic about their profession and want everybody to be as passionate about health and wellness as they are. However, "Rome was not built in a day," and small steps are often needed. Showing people how they can incorporate an effective exercise program into a busy lifestyle can go a long way toward keeping a client motivated and on the road to better health for years to come.

Exercise Intensity vs. Exercise Duration

Exercise duration refers to the time spent working out during an exercise session. *Exercise intensity* refers to how difficult or intense the workout feels. Studies show that at lower intensities of exercise, people tend to burn greater percentages of fat than at higher intensities. This has led some to believe that lower intensities of exercise are always best for fat loss. In fact, some treadmills, ellipticals, and bikes actually have a "fatburn" program that is based on this notion. On the other hand, higher intensities of exercise are associated with greater calories being used. So which is the best option to use? It turns out that both points of view have merit. When deciding which is appropriate for the client (higher intensity or longer duration), the fitness professional should always consider the initial fitness of the client. Individuals who are not accustomed to physical exertion are best served by lower intensity activity or, in the case of the very deconditioned, intermittent activity. This will allow the deconditioned individual to exercise for a longer period of time and will therefore result in a greater amount of calories being consumed. A general rule of thumb for the fitness professional should be to increase the time (duration) of activity before increasing the intensity of activity. After the individual can successfully achieve 20–60 minutes of low- to moderate-level activity with no discomfort, fitness professionals may wish to adjust the intensity of the activity to further stimulate metabolic changes.

Measuring Exercise Intensity

Exercise intensity can be measured using a variety of techniques. Not all techniques are appropriate for all people. The fitness professional must be aware of the variety of ways to measure exercise intensity and which ones are best suited for their clients. The most common techniques are listed below.

The Talk Test

The *Talk Test* is one of the simplest ways to gauge exercise intensity. The fitness professional essentially talks to the client while he or she is working out and lets the client do most of the talking. If the client can talk without undue difficulty, then exercise may be deemed well tolerated. If the client has trouble talking or cannot talk during exercise, then the intensity should be reduced to a point at which he or she can talk. This method works very well for people performing aerobic exercise and circuit training and, because it requires no math or special equipment, can be done on the fly. As such, it is popular in exercise classes.

Percent of Maximum Heart Rate

It is not uncommon for fitness professionals to prescribe a target heart rate (THR) training zone for exercise and to have clients exercise within this zone. The easiest way to assign this training zone is by first determining the client's estimated maximal number of heart beats per min (also called *estimated maximal heart rate*) and then taking percentages of this number. The determination of estimated maximum heart rate is usually achieved using the equation "220 – Age". For example, if an individual is 20 years old, he or she has an estimated maximum heart rate of 220 – 20 = 200 heart beats per minute. This means that, theoretically, the heart of a 20-year-old individual will beat no more than about 200 times in 1 minute. Now that the estimated maximum heart rate is known, percentages of this number can be calculated. Let us continue the example above and suppose that the fitness professional wanted to calculate 60% and 75% of estimated maximal heart rate:

$$200 \times 0.60 = 120 \text{ bpm}$$

$$200 \times 0.75 = 150 \text{ bpm}$$

According to this example, the person would exercise at a heart rate of between 120–150 heart beats per min (often abbreviated as bpm). This corresponds to 60% and 75%

of the person's estimated maximal ability. Any percentage that the fitness professional is looking to achieve can be estimated with this simple equation. For safety reasons, it is probably wise to start at lower percentages such as 50–65% when first working with a new client to get a better idea of how much exercise they can tolerate.

This is also important because the calculation of maximal heart rate is an estimate and thus, is not completely accurate. In fact, calculation of maximal heart rate from the "220 – Age" equation may underestimate one's true maximal heart rate.

Karvonen Heart Rate Formula

Because the "220 – Age" formula described previously is not 100% accurate, some fitness professionals opt to calculate target heart rate training zones using another method called the *Karvonen Heart Rate Formula*. This method is usually seen as more accurate than simply taking percentages of estimated maximum heart rate. To use the Karvonen formula, the resting heart rate and age of the individual must be known. The fitness professional can either measure resting heart rate him or herself after having the client rest quietly for several minutes, or they can teach their clients to measure resting heart rate themselves, preferably in the morning just after waking. The steps of the Karvonen formula are as follows:

Step 1:   220 – Age

Step 2:   Subtract resting heart rate from the result of step 1

Step 3:   Multiply the result of step 2 by percentages you wish to calculate

Step 4:   Add resting heart rate to the results of step 3

Just as before, let us examine the Karvonen method using an example:

The subject is a 30-year-old female with a resting heart rate of 60 beats per min. The fitness professional wants to calculate 60% and 80% of her maximal heart rate using the Karvonen method.

Step 1:   220 – 30 = 190 bpm

Step 2:   190 – 60 = 130 bpm

Step 3:   130 x 0.6 = 78   &   130 x 0.8 = 104

Step 4:   78 + 60 = **138**   &   104 + 60 = **164**

Answer: Target heart rate is 138 to 164 beats per minute

The ACSM generally recommends 60% and 80% when calculating target heart rate ranges for apparently healthy individuals.[1] In reality, however, fitness professionals can calculate any percentages because some people (e.g., the frail, elderly, deconditioned, etc.) may not be able to exercise aerobically at 60–80% Karvonen heart rate maximum for prolonged periods of time. When in doubt, being conservative with new clients is wise.

Ratings of Perceived Exertion

Ratings of perceived exertion (or RPE) is essentially a 0–10 scale whereby a person rates how intense they perceive their exercise exertion level to be. The other name for this method is the *Borg Scale*.

RPE Scale

Rating	Meaning
0	Nothing at all
1	Very weak effort
2	Weak effort
3	Moderately strong or difficult effort
5	Strong or difficult effort
7	Very strong or difficult effort
10	Maximal effort

Where the numbers are not in perfect order (for example, between 5 and 7), it is understood that the number that is missing would be a level of intensity in-between. For example, in the table above, level 6 is missing between level 5 and level 7. This indicates that level 6 is an exercise intensity between levels 5 and 7.

The RPE scale is very flexible and can be used to gauge difficulty during aerobic exercise ("How difficult is this level feel on a scale from 0–10?") and strength training ("How heavy does that weight feel on a 0–10 scale?"). Some even use RPE to determine fatigue level ("How tired do you feel on scale from 0–10?"). The RPE scale is also an accepted method for gauging exercise intensity in people with high blood pressure, who may be on medications that lower resting heart rate. One drawback to the RPE scale is that people must be familiar with what the numbers mean. In other words, asking somebody how they feel on a 0–10 scale will not produce an accurate result if the client has no idea what the numbers mean.

Volume of Oxygen

One of the most commonly used clinical measurements of aerobic fitness is the maximum volume of oxygen test, often abbreviated as VO_2 max. It is called "VO_2" because the letter V stands for volume and O_2 is the chemical symbol for oxygen. The

VO_2 test is a measure of how efficient we are at making energy (ATP) aerobically. As exercise intensity increases, we tend to breathe harder, taking in more oxygen, which results in an increase in VO_2. At some point during the VO_2 test, however, VO_2 will not increase as the exercise demand increases. At that point, the individual is said to have reached VO_2 max, which is the maximum volume of oxygen that can be consumed by the body to make energy aerobically. When a person is exercising at his or her VO_2 max, the individual is essentially working as hard as possible.

Most healthy individuals will have a VO_2 max of between 30–40 milliliters of oxygen per kilogram of body weight per minute. This is usually abbreviated as 30–40 ml O_2/kg BW/min. A kilogram is equal to 2.2 pounds. If we were to break a person down into kilogram increments, this means that, on average, most people would only use between 30 and 40 milliliters of oxygen per kilogram of their body their weight per minute when pushed to their absolute maximum. The VO_2 max of aerobically trained athletes tends to be higher and is generally over 50 milliliters of oxygen per kilogram of body weight per minute. While VO_2 max does have a genetic component, exercise training can result in a greater VO_2 max being achieved. The determination of VO_2 max is usually not measured in a fitness center setting. Because of the risks associated with pushing people to their absolute limit, VO_2 max is often calculated in the presence of a physician or other qualified exercise scientist and requires the use of expensive equipment. Some pieces of equipment in health clubs today, however, may make it possible to estimate the VO_2 at which a person is exercising. This brings us to the next topic, which are called METs.

Metabolic Equivalents

The term METs stands for Metabolic Equivalents. This method is based upon the fact that, at rest, every kilogram (2.2 lb.) of body weight burns 3.5 milliliters of oxygen per minute. This value of 3.5 milliliters of oxygen per kilogram of body weight per minute is referred to as 1 MET. This means that, at rest, every 2.2 pound segment of your body (that is, every kilogram of your body weight) consumes exactly 3.5 milliliters of oxygen per minute. Because of this, the intensity of activity can be described in terms of METs. For example, an activity that is 2 METs is twice as intense as resting. An activity that is 5 METs is 5 times as intense as that experienced at rest. This also means that the higher the MET level, the greater the calories consumed. Other ways to define METs include:

- 1MET = basal metabolic rate (BMR)
- 1MET= resting VO_2

Because 1 MET can also be referred to as resting VO_2 and because 1 MET is equal to 3.5 ml O_2/Kg BW/Min, this means that the number 3.5 can be used to convert METs to VO_2 and vice versa. For example, suppose someone is exercising on a treadmill at an intensity of 15 METs. Their VO_2 at that level is 15 x 3.5 = 52.5 ml O_2/Kg BW/min. Thus, METs and VO_2 are almost the same thing, just stated in different ways. Many common exercise machines in health clubs today provide estimations of METs. METs are also a common way in which medical professionals define exercise intensity.

Chapter 14

How to Read a Food Label

A central role that often remains unacknowledged in discussions about fitness professionals is that of an educator. To some individuals, one of the biggest mysteries in nutrition today sits quietly in every kitchen cabinet in America—the food label. This chapter presents an overview of the major parts of the food label in the hopes that it may assist the fitness professional to better convey nutrition information to their clients. On the following page is an example of a typical food label. For this example, a box of cereal has been chosen, but in general, all food labels have the same basic look. Let us now examine the various parts of the typical food label.

Serving Size

All food labels begin with the words "Nutrition Facts" at the top. Directly below this is the serving size that is recommended and number of servings that the package contains. By law, food labels must identify the serving size in metric units as well as in a more understandable unit of measure. In the example depicted below, we see that a serving size is 1¼ of a cup, which is equal to 30 grams. Government regulations also require that the serving size be standardized. In other words, you will not see two brands of bread or two kinds of soda with different serving sizes. Serving size is predetermined to help the consumer make easy comparisons between different brands of the same type of food. Food labels must also specify the number of servings that the package of food contains. In the example used here, the label indicates that the package contains about 13 servings. This means that if you measured all of the 1¼ cup serving sizes contained in the package, there would be about 13 servings.

Some nutrition labels contain a little trick that involves serving sizes. Nutrition labels are based on one serving only—but there may be two or more servings per container! For example, a serving size of soda is typically eight ounces, and the calories and other data on the nutrition label are based on only eight ounces, yet a 20-ounce bottle of soda contains 2 ½ servings per container. Thus, the calories and other nutrition facts on the label must be multiplied by 2.5 to arrive at the actual amounts that it contains!

NUTRITION FACTS

Serving Size 1 ¼ cup (30g)
Servings per container about 13

Amount per serving	Cereal	Cereal with ½ cup of skim milk
Calories	200	240
Calories from fat	10	10
		% Daily Value**
Total Fat 1.0g*	**2%**	**2%**
Saturated Fat 0g	0%	0%
Trans Fat 0g		
Polyunsaturated Fat 0.5		
Monounsaturated Fat 0g		
Cholesterol 0mg	0%	0%
Sodium 0mg	0%	3%
Potassium 85mg	2%	8%
Total carbohydrate 47g	16%	18%
Dietary Fiber 5g	20%	20%
Soluble Fiber less than 1 g		
Insoluble Fiber 5g		
Sugars 11g		
Protein 5g		
Vitamin A	25%	30%
Vitamin C	25%	25%
Calcium	0%	4%
Iron	2%	15%
Folate	25%	25%

*Amount in cereal
** Percent Daily Values are based on a 2,000 calorie diet.
   Your daily values may be higher or lower depending on your calorie needs.

	Calories:	2,000	2,500
Total fat	less than	65g	80g
Sat fat	less than	20g	25g
Cholesterol	less than	300mg	300mg
Sodium	less than	2,300mg	2,300mg
Potassium		3,500mg	3,500mg
Total Carbohydrate		300g	375g
Dietary Fiber		25g	30g

Calories per gram:
Fat 9   *   Carbohydrate 4   *   Protein 4

118

The serving size used in this example also tells us that we would have to eat 30 grams of this product (or 1¼ cup, if you prefer) to obtain the amount of calories, fat, carbohydrate, cholesterol, sodium, fiber, sugar, and protein listed on the label. Thus, all of the nutrient levels on the label are also based on a single serving size.

Calories

Next is the calorie content of the food. In this example, we see that the food contains 200 calories by itself and 240 calories if we consume it with ½ cup of skim milk. Directly below-calories is the number of calories from fat. Here we see that 10 calories are derived from fat if the cereal is eaten dry and 10 calories come from fat if the cereal is consumed with ½ cup of skim milk. Skim milk has negligible amounts of fat, so this is why this value does not change.

Total Fat

The total fat section of the food label indicates the total amount of fat that is contained in a serving size. In this example, the total fat is 1 gram (1 gram of fat has 9 calories, which is rounded to 10 calories in the previous section, "calories from fat"). We also see that this 1 gram of total fat represents 2% of our daily value for fat (we will discuss daily value more later). Below Total Fat are data regarding saturated, polyunsaturated, and monounsaturated fat. Trans fat is also listed on food labels because of evidence that they are linked to heart disease. Foods containing less than 1/2 gram per serving can be said to be "trans fat-free."

Cholesterol

Cholesterol must also be listed on all food labels. In the present example, we see that the food contains 0 milligrams of cholesterol per serving.

Sodium & Potassium

Just under the reference for cholesterol are listings for sodium and potassium, two other ingredients that will be listed on all food labels. In the example used here, we see that this particular food contains 0 milligrams of sodium and 85 milligrams of potassium.

Total Carbohydrate

Food labels must also indicate the total amount of carbohydrate that a serving of the food contains. In the current example, a serving contains 47 grams of carbohydrate. Total carbohydrate is an all-inclusive category and includes sugars, which are also listed separately to help people determine how much of the total carbohydrate has been contributed specifically by sugar.

Dietary Fiber

Because high-fiber diets are linked to reduced risk for various diseases, food labels list this nutrient as well. In the present example we see that a serving size contains 5 grams of fiber. Below dietary fiber are the gram amounts for both soluble (less than 1 gram) and insoluble fiber (5 grams). Both soluble and insoluble fiber appear to have different effects on the body. Soluble fiber has been shown to help lower cholesterol levels, while insoluble fiber gives food bulk and may help people feel fuller longer.

Sugar

Food labels must also list the gram amounts per serving size for sugar, which in this example is 11 grams. Unfortunately, labels do not currently tell us how much sugar is naturally occurring or is added sugars. Sugar is a simple carbohydrate and is usually listed separately from total carbohydrates. This is because all carbohydrates are not created equal. Sugars, like table sugar, tend to raise blood glucose levels quickly and generally do not contain many nutrients. Complex carbohydrates are more nutrient-dense and raise blood glucose levels more slowly. Thus, they are considered to be healthier than simple sugars. It is possible to have a lot of carbohydrates yet have few or even 0 grams of sugar in a food. Notice also that there is no daily value listed for sugars. This is because sugar does not have any specific recommendations for intake. This is contrasted from the "total carbohydrate" section, which does have a daily value.

Protein

Keeping track of how much protein somebody eats is pretty simple because all food labels list this amount. In the present example, the food label indicates 5 grams of protein per serving. There is no RDA for protein.

Vitamins and Minerals

By law, food labels must list the percent daily values for vitamin A, vitamin C, calcium, and iron. Other vitamins and minerals may also be listed on the food label, although this is not mandatory.

What Are Daily Values?

Most who read food labels have probably noticed a lot of percentages for the different nutrients. These are the daily values (DVs). Daily values represent suggested nutrient intake levels that are appropriate for most individuals, regardless of age or gender. For example, on the food label used here, we see that each serving of product contains 47 grams of carbohydrate and that this represents 16% of our daily value for this nutrient. The daily values—which are based on the RDAs—were adopted because RDAs can fluctuate according to age and gender as well as other conditions. Thus, daily values are meant to help make reading food labels easier. The daily values listed for the nutrients on food labels are based a 2,000-calorie-per-day diet. Close to the bottom of food labels you will also see the daily values for several nutrients listed for someone consuming a 2,500-calorie-per-day diet. Both 2,000- and 2,500-calorie diets were chosen so as to make the food label more applicable to the diets of most Americans. In other words, the reasoning was that most Americans consume somewhere between 2,000 and 2,500 calories per day. Below are the daily values of some of the most important nutrients. These values are listed at the bottom of most food labels as well.

Daily Values (Based on a 2000 calorie diet)	
Nutrient	Daily Value
Total Fat	65 grams
Saturated Fat	20 grams
Cholesterol	300 milligrams
Total Carbohydrate	300 grams
Dietary Fiber	25 grams
Sodium	2300 milligrams
Potassium	3500 milligrams
Protein	50 grams

Calories per Gram

At the very bottom of most food labels are the calories that are contained in a gram of fat, carbohydrate, and protein (9, 4, and 4 calories, respectively). These numbers can be used to calculate the actual number of calories from fat, carbohydrate, and protein in a serving size of the food in question. For example, on the food label used here, we see that the total carbohydrate in one serving is 47 grams. Since each gram of carbohydrate contains 4 calories, this means that 47 x 4 = 188 calories from carbohydrate in one serving. If we wanted to know what percent of the food was carbohydrate, we would divide the calories from carbohydrates (188) by the total calories in a serving (200). This would equal 188 ÷ 200 = 94% carbohydrate. Thus, the food in this example is composed of about 94% carbohydrate per serving. These same calculations can be done for fat and protein.

Food Label Buzz Words

In the past, food labels could list almost anything. This is no longer the case, as the regulations that govern what can and cannot be claimed on food labels are very specific. What follows is a summary of the major allowable food label claims and what they mean.

- **Fat Free.** In order for a product to post the label that its "fat free," it must either have 0 grams of fat or contain an insignificant amount of fat (usually defined as less than ½ gram per serving).

- **Low Fat.** Foods that make the claim that they are "low fat" can only do so if they contain less than 3 grams of fat per serving size.

- **Low in Saturated Fat.** A food that is low in saturated fat must contain less than 1 gram of saturated fat per serving.

- **Cholesterol Free.** To be called cholesterol free, the food in question must contain less than 2 milligrams of cholesterol per serving size.

- **Calorie Free.** By law, only foods that contain fewer than 5 calories per serving can make the calorie-free claim. Therefore, even calorie-free foods technically have some calories.

- **Sodium Free.** Foods listed as sodium free can only do so if they contain less than 2 milligrams of sodium per serving.

- **Light (or Lite).** For a food package to make the claim that it is light, it must contain either 1/3 fewer calories or 1/2 the amount of fat as the original recipe of the product. Beware—it is possible for a food to make this claim yet still contain high amounts of fat. For example, suppose the original recipe had 99 grams of fat and the light version has 1/3 less. That means that the light version has 66 grams of fat—the entire daily value for fat! Here is a good rule of thumb: do the math yourself when you see this claim.

- **Healthy.** For a product to use the word "healthy," it must provide at least 10% of the daily value per serving of any or all of the following: vitamin A, vitamin C, calcium, iron, fiber, or protein. In addition, each serving must contain no more than 60 mg of cholesterol and no more than 480 mg sodium.

- **Good Source.** A food can be labeled a "good source" of various nutrients if the food contains between 10–19% more than the daily value of the nutrient in question. In addition, there must be scientific evidence showing that the nutrient in question has health benefits. For example, evidence suggests that folate can lower birth defects. Thus, foods high in folate can be said to be a good source of this vitamin. If there is no proof of health benefits associated with elevated levels of a nutrient, then the "good source" claim cannot be made. Other terms for "good source" that also show up on food labels include "high," "rich in," and "excellent source."

- **Reduced.** For a food label to make the "reduced" claim, it must contain at least 25% fewer calories, fat, saturated fat, cholesterol, sodium, or sugar than the original recipe for the product. Thus, if the original recipe had 100 grams of total fat, then the "reduced" claim could be made if the new version of the product had 75 grams of fat per serving.

- **Organic.** According the USDA, the term "organic" means that a food was grown without the use of synthetic fertilizers, biotechnology, or radiation. Most pesticides are also banned from being used with organic foods. In 2002, the US Department of Agriculture launched its official federal guidelines regarding when foods may call themselves "organic." According to these guidelines, three terms may now be displayed on foods. The terms and their definitions are found below.

  - **"100% organic"** means that all of a product's ingredients are organic.

  - **"Organic"** is different than 100% organic and means that at least 95% of a product's ingredients are organic.

  - **"Made with Organic Ingredients"** means that the product has at least 70% organically derived ingredients.

- **Natural.** Despite showing up frequently on food labels, the word "natural" has no legal definition. As such, it carries much less weight than "organic," "healthy," or other words mentioned in this section. In theory, a food that only bears the "natural" label could be high in saturated fat, trans fat, or other compounds that most people associate with being unhealthy.

Chapter 15

Questions & Answers

Fitness professionals are always being asked questions about health, wellness, exercise, and about how to make sense of health reports appearing in magazines, on TV, and on the internet. This chapter is about not only these questions, but also questions that fitness professionals themselves may be asking while continuing to struggle with finding straight answers.

Q. How much protein do I need?
A. It is different for different people. Many studies suggest that as a general rule with exercise, a protein range of between about 0.6 grams per pound to about 0.9 grams per pound is ideal. Some round up to 1 gram per pound, but this may be too much for those who do a significant amount of cardio. Protein intake should be spread throughout the day as opposed to having it all at once.

Q. Someone told me that they are not allowed to eat grapefruit. Why?
A. This is probably because grapefruit can interfere with an enzyme involved in the breakdown of different types of prescription medications. This can interfere with how well the medication works. In some books, this is called the "grapefruit effect."

Q. After a workout, my urine looks like "iced tea." What is that?
A. Darkly colored urine (the color of iced tea or cola) may be a sign of a condition called rhabdomyolysis, which occurs from the breakdown of muscle tissue. This is a very serious medical disorder that can be caused by many things, including doing too much exercise. "Rhabdo," as it is also called, can result in kidney failure. It can also cause swelling of the limbs and extreme muscle pain. People who suspect that they have this condition need to seek medical help immediately. For more information, see my article *"Rhabdomyolysis and Personal Training: Facts You Need To Know,"* found at my website, www.Joe-Cannon.com. There, I cover this condition in greater detail. Fitness trainers need to know about this condition.

Q. What is gluten?
A. Gluten is a protein found in products containing wheat, rye, or barley. As such, it shows up frequently in the foods that we eat. People with the digestive disorder celiac disease have a problem digesting gluten. In these people (which could be 1 in every 133 Americans), gluten provokes the immune system, which then inflames and damages the small intestine, causing gastrointestinal distress. Some research links celiac disease with the development of type I diabetes, rheumatoid arthritis, and other

disorders. After celiac disease is diagnosed by a physician, the person should avoid foods that contain gluten.

Q. How do people lose weight on low-carb diets?

A. When a person starts a low-carbohydrate diet, they will likely lose a large amount of weight within the first couple of weeks. The main reason for this has to do with glycogen, which is the body's storage form of sugar. When we significantly reduce the amount of carbohydrates we eat, our body begins to degrade its glycogen reserves in order to keep our blood sugar from falling too much (we can die if blood sugar gets to low!). As glycogen is utilized, a lot of water is released in the process. In fact, for every gram of glycogen that is used, roughly 3 grams of water are freed up! The body has to do something with all of that water, so it sends people to the bathroom to get rid of it. Thus, for the first few weeks, most of the weight lost on a low-carb diet is in the form of water. Another reason why these diets lead to weight loss is because a limited variety of foods is eaten. Research shows that people eat more when they have a variety of foods from which to choose than when there are fewer choices. Cutting carbs reduces the number of choices on these diets. This cuts out additional calories and probably leads to further weight loss. Also see my blog post, "Low Carb diets: How They Really Work" Dat Joe-Cannon.com.

Q. What is a normal cholesterol level?

A. Currently, a total cholesterol level of less than 200 mg/dL is considered normal and healthy for adults. In addition, people should strive for their LDL to be less than 100 mg/dL. Triglycerides should be less than 150 mg/dL. With respect to HDL, greater than 40 mg/dL is advisable. In fact, an HDL of 60 mg/dL or more is often called a "negative risk factor" for heart disease (that is, it reduces heart disease risk). While weight loss often can sometimes improve cholesterol levels, exercise, especially aerobic exercise, helps raise HDL levels.

Q. Is flax better than fish oil?

A. Both flax seeds and fish oil contain omega-3 fatty acids, which some studies show are "heart-healthy." However, they do not contain the same types of omega-3s. Flax contains alpha-linolenic acid (ALA), while fish oil has EPA and DHA. We have a very limited ability to convert ALA into EPA and DHA. Both types of fatty acids are healthy, but their effects may not be the same. As such, it is best to ingest both through the diet rather than focusing on only one of them.

Q. What is the difference between an RD and a nutritionist?

A. A registered dietitian (RD) is someone who has at least a BS degree in nutrition and has passed the American Dietetics Association certification test. Most also do an internship under the tutelage of another qualified dietitian. A nutritionist is a more general term that may or may not refer to an RD. Some dietitians do refer to themselves as nutritionists. However, depending on the state in which one resides, the term "nutritionist" might be used by almost anyone—including those with no formal nutrition education or certification.

Q. Can personal trainers give nutrition advice?

A. Laws may differ from state to state. Fitness professionals are encouraged to visit their local county government or consult a legal professional for the laws in their area. For those who work at health clubs, additional rules may also apply. Some health clubs may have specific staff associates to whom they refer members for nutrition-related information. Regardless of issues of legality and internal health club policies, fitness professionals should strive to network with nutrition professionals like registered dietitians (RDs). Dietitians undoubtedly have clients who are trying to lose weight and who need to exercise. Likewise, personal trainers usually have a number of clients whom they could refer to a dietician for help with nutrition. Generally, dietitians know nutrition but not exercise technique. This is a void that an alliance with a personal trainer could fill very well. Also see my post, "Personal Trainers And Nutrition Advice: Yes or No" at Joe-Cannon.com, where I go into greater detail on this issue.

Q. Can personal trainers recommend supplements?

A. I believe that trainers need to be careful about supplements that they recommend and sell. Trainers have been sued because of supplements, and some personal trainer insurance policies will not protect trainers if a lawsuit occurs. Trainers should not assume that something labeled "natural" is safe for everybody. This is especially true for people who have medical issues or who take medications. I believe that trainers need to be especially cautious of "fat burners" and herbal supplements. For more on supplements, see my site, Supplement-Geek.com. Also read my post *"Should Personal Trainers Recommend Supplements?"* at www.Joe-Cannon.com to learn more about why I recommend using caution with this issue.

Q. Can people lose fat in only certain areas?

A. Unfortunately, with the exception of liposuction, it is not possible to lose fat from only specific areas of the body. This fallacy is referred to as "spot reduction" and, ironically, is the premise behind many weight loss gizmos advertised on TV. If spot reduction worked, one would expect to see less fat on the dominant arm of a tennis player or a baseball pitcher, as these athletes typically exercise one limb more than the other. However, this is not what is observed. Rather, when we exercise, we lose fat all over the body at the same time. Thus, we lose fat from under our arms, on our thighs and tummies, around our internal organs, and even from our little pinky fingers! Overall, this is a far healthier way to lose excess body fat.

Q. What does partially hydrogenated mean?

A. To hydrogenate a fat means to add hydrogen atoms to it. This changes the chemical properties of the fat. Saturated fats are literally saturated with hydrogen atoms. Partially hydrogenated, while less saturated with hydrogen than fully hydrogenated fat, is nevertheless a saturated fat as well. Another phrase that is often used on food labels is "tropical oils." Tropical oils such as palm oil, palm kernel oil, and coconut oil are also saturated fats. Saturated fats are implicated in the development of heart disease and should therefore be avoided as much as possible. Specifically, saturated fats have been shown to raise LDL (bad cholesterol). Considering how harmful these fats are, some might wonder why they are used in the first place. One reason is that saturated fats help increase the shelf life of a food, which in turn keeps the price down. Think about how expensive cookies and cakes might be if they spoiled after a few days! Therefore, from an economical viewpoint, saturated fats make sense, but from a health viewpoint, they are things to avoid. While partially hydrogenated fats contain fewer hydrogen atoms, they are likely to possess more trans fats, which were discussed earlier in this book.

Q. What are sugar alcohols?
A. While technically neither a sugar nor an alcohol, sugar alcohols are molecules that look like both sugars and alcohols. Because they tend to contain fewer calories than regular sugar (1.5–3 calories per gram as opposed to 4 calories per gram for sugar), sugar alcohols are often used in place of sugar in low-calorie and low-carb foods as well as in some nutritional supplements. Common sugar alcohols include mannitol, sorbitol, and xylitol. Another difference between traditional carbohydrates and sugar alcohols is that sugar alcohols do not raise insulin levels very much, if at all. Thus, sugar alcohols may also be found in diabetic foods. Sugar alcohols do not contain any alcohol like the kind found in alcoholic beverages, so they will not make people drunk.

Q. What does the "L" on amino acid supplement labels mean?
A. The letter "L" that is on the labels of amino acid supplements is a chemistry term meaning that the molecules are "left handed." Molecules, like people, can be either right-handed or left-handed. It turns out that all essential and non-essential amino acids in the human body are left-handed. As a result, amino acids are given names like L arginine, L glutamine, and others.

Q. Is olive oil responsible for the effects of the Mediterranean Diet?
A. The words "olive oil" and "Mediterranean diet" are used together so often that it is easy for people to think that all they have to do is add olive oil to foods to reap the benefits of this eating style. I believe that this is missing the big picture. The Mediterranean diet includes fruits, vegetables, whole gains, and fish. People often like to drill diets down to a single ingredient (like olive oil) to explain observed benefits, but this does not always work out well. It is very likely that the power of the Mediterranean diet to reduce heart disease risk has less to do with olive oil than it has to do with all of the other healthy foods that it incorporates.

Q. Do we have to exercise for 20 minutes before burning fat?
A. The statement that we must exercise for 20–30 minutes before we begin to use our fat reserves is popular in fitness. In reality, however, we are always burning fat, it is just a matter of how much we are talking about. At rest, roughly 60% of the energy burned come from fat, while about 40% stems from carbohydrate burning. When exercise starts, we begin to burn more carbs and less fat. However, as we continue to exercise, a gradual shift occurs at which we begin using fewer carbs and more fat. So, do we have to exercise for at lest 20 minutes before we start the fat burning process? Technically, no, but after 20 minutes of exercise, we are using a lot more fat than we do after only 1 minute of exercise. Also, the longer one exercises, the more calories he or she burns.

Q. Can we drink too much water?

A. Yes. A condition exists in which individuals consume so much water during exercise that they may suffer life-threatening symptoms. This condition is called *hyponatremia* (pronounced "hypo-nay-tree-me-ah"). Hyponatremia results when water is consumed in such excess that it dilutes the concentration of the body's sodium and other electrolytes. Remember that sodium (along with potassium) plays a major role in facilitating both muscle contraction and the transmission of nerve impulses. Sodium is also responsible for keeping the body's fluid levels at their proper concentrations. As fluid levels increase (by drinking water), the concentration of sodium and other electrolytes actually decreases as it is dispersed through a greater volume of fluid. This, coupled with sodium losses through sweat, can lead to life-threatening consequences. Some evidence suggests that the body can only eliminate about 1 quart of water per hour. Thus, consuming 2 or more quarts per hour during exercise could, in theory, lead to hyponatremia.

While typically observed in those who compete in long-endurance events like marathons and triathlons, hyponatremia may also occur in other events such as football. This is particularly true during pre-season training for sports, when the individual may not be accustomed to the rigors of exercise and may be more likely to consume large volumes of water. Hyponatremia requires immediate medical attention, and treatment involves intravenous sodium replacement. Symptoms of hyponatremia include swollen feet and hands, nausea, vomiting, and confusion or disorientation, to name a few. One possible sign that hyponatremia may occur is weight gain immediately following exercise. Normally, one would expect to lose weight after exercise due to fluid losses from sweat. Weight gain immediately after exercise may indicate that the person has consumed too much water. While this observation is not foolproof, noticing weight gain after exercise may allow the fitness professional an opportunity to discuss hyponatremia with his or her clients. The goal here is not to frighten individuals to not drink any water, but rather to make them aware of a situation that may occur with excessive fluid consumption.

Q. Are natural vitamins better than synthetic vitamins?

A. Technically, the body does not know the difference between synthetic vitamins made in the laboratory and natural vitamins made in nature. This is because the chemical structures of synthetic and natural vitamins are identical.

The case for vitamin E is one classic example often used in an attempt to prove the superiority of natural over synthetic vitamins. It turns out that the body does, in fact, utilize natural vitamin E more efficiently than synthetic vitamin E—and for a very good reason. Some people in the world are left-handed while others are right-handed. The same is also true for molecules! Technically, we refer to left-handed molecules as levorotory (or "L" for short), while right-handed molecules are given the name dextrorotatory (or "d" for short). The human body prefers right-handed (d) vitamin E over left-hand (L) vitamin E. So in theory, natural vitamin E would be composed of all right-handed molecules (in other words, only the d version). Synthetic vitamin E is actually composed of a mixture of both right- and left-handed molecules (referred to as "dl alpha tocopherol" on many multivitamin labels). However, we can only use the right-handed

(d) version. Theoretically, then, only 50% of synthetic vitamin E can be utilized by the body. It should be noted, however, that right-handed vitamin E made in the laboratory is absorbed no differently than right-handed vitamin E made in nature's laboratory.

Q. With creatine supplements, is the "loading phase" needed?
A. When creatine first came to public attention, everybody was advocating that people begin with what was called a "loading phase" whereby 20–25 grams per day of creatine would be used for the first week of supplementation. This was then to be followed by a "maintenance phase" that consisted of only 2–5 grams per day. Is the loading phase needed to reap the benefits of creatine? Apparently it is not. In a study published in the *Journal of Applied Physiology*, researchers found that 28 days of using 3 grams of creatine per day enhanced muscle creatine reserves as effectively as 20 grams per day for a week.[129] The take home message seems clear—if you are not in a hurry, loading creatine is not needed. For more on creatine, read my book entitled *Nutritional Supplements*, available at my website www.Joe-Cannon.com. Also, see the creatine section of Supplement-Geek.com.

Q. When is the best time to take multivitamins?
A. While there is no "best" or perfect time to take multivitamins, as a general rule, it is probably best to take multivitamins with food. This is because when you eat, you produce more stomach acid, which helps with vitamin absorption. In addition, because a meal probably contains some fat, this will also help with the absorption of the fat soluble vitamins (A, E, D, and K) as well.

Q. What is better—protein before or after exercise?
A. Both strategies have merit. Eating some protein (and carbs) 2–3 hrs before a workout can help supply the body with nutrients needed during training. That said, this practice might cause cramping or GI problems for some, especially for those who eat a big meal just prior to exercise. Research also suggests that consuming protein (and carbs) as soon as possible (i.e., within 1 hour) after exercise appears to be better for building muscle than eating several hours after exercise.[141] Still other research states that it doesn't matter. While for healthy people it may not matter as much when they eat, this issue may be important for older adults dealing with sarcopenia.

For the answers to over 100 other questions, see "*Personal Trainers Big Book of Questions And Answers*", found at www.Joe-Cannon.com.

Glossary

Adipose Tissue. Adipose is another name for fat tissue. Triglycerides are stored in adipose tissue.

Aerobic Exercise. Exercise that uses oxygen as a means to generate energy (ATP). Also, any exercise that one can perform for a prolonged period of time without stopping. Usually, during aerobic exercise, fat is used as a fuel source. Examples include walking, swimming, bike riding, and jogging.

AI. A nutrition term which stands for "adequate intake." Adequate intakes for nutrients are used by nutrition professionals when there is not enough evidence available for an RDA to be determined. See also *RDA* and *UL*.

Amenorrhea. The cessation of menstrual cycles. May occur with anorexia nervosa. See also *oligomenorrhea*.

Amino Acid. The building blocks of proteins. There are 20 amino acids that the body uses to make proteins. Amino acids can be divided into essential (which we must obtain from food) and non-essential (which our bodies can make on their own) amino acids. See also *proteins*.

Anabolism. Refers to the buildup or synthesis of substances in the body. See also *catabolism*.

Anaerobic Exercise. Exercise that does not require oxygen to help with the generation of energy (ATP). Examples are weight lifting, powerlifting, and sprinting.

Antioxidant. Any substance that reduces the production of free radicals. Vitamins E and C are classic examples of antioxidants. See also *free radical*.

ATP. Adenosine Triphosphate. ATP is the body's ultimate energy molecule. ATP is an immediate source of energy for muscle contraction. The energy (calories) in food is rearranged into a usable form of energy—ATP.

Bioelectric Impedance Analysis. A method of body composition determination that uses a small electric current that passes through the body. Sometimes abbreviated "BIA." See also *hydrostatic weighing*.

BMR. Basal Metabolic Rate. The lowest metabolism possible. See also *RMR*.

Body Composition. The amount of fat and fat-free mass that a body contains.

Body Mass Index. A relatively quick way to assess body composition. Abbreviated "BMI." BMI is equal to a person's weight in kilograms divided by height in meters squared (BMI = weight (kg) ÷ height (m^2)). As BMI increases, so, too, does risk for obesity-related disease.

Calorie. A calorie is a unit of heat energy. Specifically, it is the amount of heat needed to raise 1 kilogram of water (1 liter) 1 degree Celsius. Calories are the key to weight loss and weight gain. Consuming more calories than are expended through exercise and daily activities results in weight gain. Consuming fewer calories than are expended through exercise and daily activities results in weight loss. Calories are derived from the three macronutrients— proteins, carbohydrates, and fats. Other synonymous names for calorie include "kilogram calorie," "Kcal," and kilocalorie.

Carbohydrate. Carbohydrates are sugars. Carbohydrates are the primary energy source used during exercise. Every gram of carbohydrate has 4 calories. Food sources of carbohydrates include breads, cereals, pasta, rice, etc.

Cardiovascular Exercise. Any exercise that one can do for a prolonged period of time without stopping. Examples include walking, hiking, jogging, swimming, and bike riding. It is also called "aerobic exercise."

Catabolism. Refers to the breaking down of a substance in the body. See also *anabolism.*

Cholesterol. A substance made in the liver that is indispensable for life. Too much, though, can build up in the body and eventually contribute to diseases such as high blood pressure, strokes, and heart attacks. See also *HDL* and *LDL cholesterol.*

Complete Protein. Also called high-quality protein. A complete protein source contains all of the essential amino acids in the proper amounts for humans. Meats, poultry, and fish are good sources of complete proteins.

Creatine Phosphate. Creatine is an energy source that the body uses to regenerate ATP during periods of intense physical activity like sprinting or heavy weight lifting. Creatine is found in meat and fish products and is also naturally produced in the body.

Diabetes. A disease in which the body either does not make insulin or cannot make use of the insulin that is present. Diabetes is divided into Type I, in which the person does not make insulin (so insulin must be injected daily) and Type II, in which the individual cannot make use of the insulin that is made. Overweight individuals are at risk for both types of diabetes.

Dietary Supplement. Defined as any substance for use by man to supplement the diet by increasing the total dietary intake. Includes, but is not limited to, vitamins, minerals, herbs, some hormones, amino acids, and enzymes.

DNA. Stands for "de-oxy-ribo-nucleic acid." Our genetic material. DNA is a "blueprint" or "software program" of how to make another you. The chromosomes are made of DNA.

DRI. Dietary reference intake. A nutrition term that was created when the RDA was revamped.

Enzyme. A biological catalyst. Enzymes are biological "machines" that speed up chemical reactions and help them occur more quickly than they normally would. Practically every chemical reaction in the body requires an enzyme. Enzymes are manufactured in the body and can be used over again many times before wearing out. When an enzyme finally wears out, an identical enzyme is made.

Ephedra. Ephedra is the herb that contains the drug ephedrine, which mimics the effect of adrenaline in the body. Also called "Ma-Huang." Side effects of ephedra can include increased heart rate and blood pressure and possibly death.

Ergogenic Aid. Ergogenic aids may be any substance or product that is touted to enhance exercise ability. Examples of ergogenic aids include creatine, caffeine, androstendione, and even some clothing products, to name a few.

Essential. In reference to nutrition, "essential" refers to a substance that must be consumed in the diet. For example, essential amino acids are "essential" because we cannot make them and must therefore obtain them from food or supplements.

Fat. Fat is the body's long-term energy storage molecule. Every gram of fat has 9 calories. In contrast, protein and carbohydrate only have about 4 calories per gram. One pound of fat contains 3,500 calories.

Fiber. The name given to indigestible carbohydrates derived from plants. Fiber can be subdivided into soluble fiber and insoluble fiber.

Free Radical. A molecule or atom that can disrupt normal cellular functioning. Free radicals are produced by normal cellular activities and are normally kept in check by antioxidant defense systems as well as by foods that contain antioxidants. In excess, however, it is theorized that free radicals may contribute to a wide variety of diseases and syndromes such as cancer. It is not possible to completely rid the body of free radicals. See also *antioxidant.*

Gene. A region of DNA that contains genetic instructions for specific traits such as eye color, muscle fiber type, or bone density. See also *DNA.*

Glucose. Blood sugar. Normal blood sugar is < 100 mg/dL. See also *glycogen* and *glycolysis.*

Glycogen. Storage form of carbohydrate. Glycogen is made up of sugar (glucose). The body stores a certain amount of sugar for use during exercise and during periods of non-eating. This sugar is called glycogen. It is from this term that we get the word "glycolysis." See also *glycolysis.*

Glycolysis. The chemical pathway responsible for the breakdown of sugar (glucose) for energy (ATP) that does not require oxygen. Glycolysis is an anaerobic energy generating pathway. Generally, as exercise intensity increases, so does glycolysis. A byproduct of glycolysis is lactic acid, which causes a burning sensation inside the muscles as well as muscle fatigue. See also *ATP, glycogen* and *glucose.*

Gram. Unit of weight in the metric system. There are about 28 grams in 1 ounce. See also *protein, fat* and *carbohydrate.*

HDL. The so-called "good" cholesterol. HDL (high density lipoprotein) is a molecule that transports cholesterol. HDL transports cholesterol from the blood back to the liver, where it is broken down. It is advantageous to have a high level of HDL in the blood in light of evidence that HDL can help reduce the risk of heart disease. On blood tests, HDL should be 40 mg/dL or better. See also *LDL* and *cholesterol.*

Hormone. A chemical messenger. The body contains many hormones such as testosterone, estrogen, and insulin. Hormones regulate many biological processes.

Hydrogenation. The process of making a saturated fat from an unsaturated fat. During the hydrogenation process, a fat is saturated with hydrogen atoms. High intakes of saturated fats are linked to heart disease. See also *saturated* and *unsaturated fat.*

Hypercholesterolemia. Another name for high cholesterol levels. See also *cholesterol, HDL* and *LDL.*

Hypertension. High blood pressure. Hypertension is blood pressure that is chronically above 140/90 mm Hg. The letters "mm Hg" stand for millimeters of mercury. Hypertension is sometimes abbreviated as "HTN." Hypertension places one at greater risk for heart disease.

Insulin. A hormone made within the beta cells of the pancreas. It lowers blood sugar.

Ketone. A molecule formed during severe calorie or carbohydrate restriction. Ketones can act as an alternative energy source for many of the body's cells. Excessive ketone formation (ketosis) is dangerous in that it alters the chemistry of the body (i.e., decreases pH, which increases acidity of the body). This, in turn, negatively affects normal body functions. See also *pH.*

Kilogram. A metric system unit of measurement. One kilogram = 1,000 grams. One kilogram (or 1 kg) is equal to about 2.2 pounds.

Krebs Cycle. The name given to the chemical reaction that involves the aerobic breakdown of fat. The Krebs cycle occurs in the mitochondria. Other names for the Krebs cycle include the "TCA cycle" (tricarboxylic acid cycle) and the "citric acid cycle." See also *mitochondria, fat, carbohydrate,* and *glycolysis.*

Lactic Acid. A metabolic byproduct of glycolysis made during the anaerobic breaking down sugar (glucose) for energy (ATP). Elevations in lactic acid alter the pH of cells and cause the burning sensation in muscles during intense exercise.

LDL. The so-called "bad" cholesterol. LDL (low density lipoprotein) is a molecule that transports cholesterol. LDL transports cholesterol from where it is made out to the cells of the body, where it can be used. High levels of LDL in the blood are deemed a contributor to heart disease.

Lean Body Mass. Traditionally, lean body mass (LBM) has been used to refer to muscle mass. Lean body mass, however, may be anything in the body other than fat mass. Thus, LBM also includes bone and water.

Lipid. Another name for fat.

Macronutrient. Nutrients that make up the greatest amount of our diet. Proteins, fats, and carbohydrates are the macronutrients. See also *protein, fat,* and *carbohydrate.*

MET. Stands for "metabolic equivalents." One MET is equal to 3.5 milliliters of oxygen per kilogram of body weight per minute. METs are another way to measure exercise intensity. An exercise intensity of 3 METs is 3 times more difficult as an intensity of 1 MET. See also *oxygen consumption* and VO_2.

Metabolic syndrome. Pre-diabetes.

Metabolism. The total of all of the building-up chemical reactions (anabolic reactions) and breaking-down chemical reactions (catabolic reactions) in the body. Metabolism can also be thought of as the speed at which we burn calories. Faster metabolisms burn calories faster than slower metabolisms.

Mitochondria. A region of the cell where fat is broken down to generate energy (ATP). Aerobic exercise can stimulate production of more mitochondria. See also *fat* and *Krebs cycle*.

Non-Essential. With regard to nutrition, a substance that does not need to be obtained from food or supplements. In other words, the body can produce the substance on its own. Non-essential amino acids are examples of non-essential nutrients. See also *amino acid*.

Oligomenorrhea. Irregular menstrual cycles. May be observed in bulimia nervosa. See also *amenorrhea*.

Osteoporosis. A disease in which bones become brittle and break easily. Osteoporosis can affect not only women, but men also. Bone loss begins around the age of 35.

Peer-Reviewed. A scientific study is peer-reviewed when it is first reviewed by other competent scientists (peers) prior to publication. This decreases errors that might have occurred in the study and allows for a better study. Articles printed in popular magazines and newspapers are generally not peer-reviewed.

pH. Refers to an acidity scale that is commonly used in science. The scale runs from 0–14. A pH of 7 is considered neutral. The lower the number on the pH scale, the more acidic a substance is. Overall, the pH of the human body is about 7.35.

Phosphagen. A high energy-containing molecule. ATP and phosphocreatine are examples of the phosphagens.

Phytonutrients. Nutrients derived from fruits and vegetables. Also called "phytochemicals."

Protein. One of the macronutrients. Protein contains 4 calories per gram. Proteins are made of smaller units called amino acids. See also *amino acid*.

RDA. Recommended Dietary Allowance. The RDAs represent nutrient intakes in amounts needed to ward off diseases associated with nutrient deficiencies.

Registered Dietitian. A registered dietitian (RD) is a nutrition professional who has at least a bachelor's degree in nutrition and who has passed the American Dietetic Association (ADA) examination.

Rhabdomyolysis. A serious medical condition that is caused by the breakdown of skeletal muscle fibers. See www.Joe-Cannon.com for more information about exercise-induced rhabdomyolysis.

RMR. Resting Metabolic Rate. The minimum number of calories needed to sustain the vital functions of the body. RMR is proportional to body size. Thus, taller, heavier people have a higher RMR than do shorter, lighter people. Resting metabolic rate tends to decrease by 2–5% per decade after age 40. *BMR*.

Sarcopenia. Muscle loss that occurs during the aging process.

Saturated Fat. A saturated fat is saturated with hydrogen atoms. Saturated fats are less healthy than unsaturated fats. Saturated fats tend to be solid at room temperature.

Sedentary. A term that refers to minimal physical activity.

Thermogenic. Relates to raising metabolic rate or burning calories.

Trans Fatty Acid. Refers to the molecular arrangement of the atoms that make up a fat. Trans fatty acids are usually made when saturated fats are made. Research shows that some trans fatty acids may be detrimental to health by fostering heart disease. See also *saturated fat, unsaturated fat, HDL, LDL* and *cholesterol.*

Triglyceride. Another name for fat. Triglycerides are stored in fat cells and are released into the blood when needed, such as during aerobic exercise. See also *adipose tissue.*

UL. A nutrition term that stands for "tolerable upper intake level." It refers to the highest level of a nutrient that can be safely consumed. Intakes above the UL increase the potential that negative side effects might occur. See also *AI, DRI* and *RDA.*

Unsaturated Fat. Unsaturated fats tend to be liquid at room temperature and are heart-healthy. Unsaturated fats are not as saturated with hydrogen atoms as saturated fats. Monounsaturated fats and polyunsaturated fats refer to the degree of saturation. See also *saturated fat.*

Vitamin. An organic substance needed in small amounts by the body to help sustain life processes. Vitamins can be divided into water-soluble vitamins (B complex and vitamin C) and fat-soluble vitamins (A, D, E, and K). See also *mineral.*

VO_2. Abbreviation for "volume of oxygen." VO_2 is used as a measure of exercise intensity and aerobic fitness. See also *oxygen consumption* and *METs.*

References

1. ACSM Position Stand (2001). Appropriate intervention strategies for weight loss and prevention of weight regain in adults Medicine and Science in Sports and Exercise, 33, 12, 2145-2156.
2. ACSM (2000). ACSM's Guidelines for Exercise Testing and Prescription, 6th edition. Lippincott, Williams and Wilkins.
3. ACSM Position Stand (1997). Female Athletic Triad. Medicine and Science in Sports and Exercise, 29, 5, pp. i-ix.
4. Adebowale, A. O. et al. (2000). Analysis of glucosamine and chondroitin sulfate content in marketed products and the caco-2 permeability of chondroitin sulfate raw materials. Journal of the American Nutraceutical Association,3, 1, 37-44.
5. Alexander, J. L. (2002). The role of resistance exercise in weight loss. Strength & Conditioning Journal, 24, 11, 65-69.
6. Arner, P. et al. (1990). Expression of lipoprotein lipase in different human subcutaneous adipose tissue regions. Journal of Lipid Research, 32, 423-430.
7. Bachle, L. et al. (2001). The effect of fluid replacement on endurance performance. Journal of Strength and Conditioning Research, 15, 2, 217-224.
8. Ballantyne, C. S. et al. (2000). The acute effects of androstenedione supplementation in healthy young males. Canadian Journal of Applied Physiology, 25, 1, 68-78.
9. Ballor, D. L. et al. (1994). Exercise training enhances fat-free mass preservation during diet-induced weight loss: a meta-analytical finding. International Journal of Obesity, 18, 35-43.
10. Baulieu, E. (1996). Dehydroepiandrosterone (DHEA): A fountain of youth? Journal of Clinical Endocrinology and Metabolism, 81, 9, 3147-3151.
11. Bloomfield, S. A. (1997). Osteoporosis. In: ACSM's Exercise Management for Persons with Chronic Diseases and Disabilities. Human Kinetics.
12. Bonci, L. (2003). Let 'em eat lettuce. Training & Conditioning, 13, 3, 31-36.
13. Brandsch, C. et al. (2002). Effect of L-carnitine on weight loss and body composition of rats fed a hypocaloric diet. Annals of Nutrition and Metabolism, 46, 5,205-210.
14. Brownell, K. D. et al. (1986). The effects of repeated cycles of weight loss and regain in rats. Physiology and Behavior, 35, 459-465.
15. Casa, J. et al. (2000). Journal of Athletic Training, 35, 2, 212-224.
16. Cerny,F. J. Burton, H.W. (2001). Exercise Physiology for Health Care Professionals, Human Kinetics.
17. Clark, N. (2001). Nutrition in Action: How to Fuel Your Body for Sports & Health. A PowerPoint presentation. Human Kinetics.
18. Clarkson, P. (2001). Supplements containing ephedrine: are they safe and do they work? Gatorade Sports Science Institute. http://www.gssiweb.com/
19. da Camara, C. C. (1998). Glucosamine sulfate for osteoarthritis. Annals of Pharmacotherapy, 32, 580-587.
20. DeGroot, L. J. (1995). Endocrinology, 3rd edition. Volume 3. W.B. Saunders.
21. Dolins, K. R. (2002). Sports nutrition for the endurance athlete. Presented at: Inside the Athlete: Fueling the Athlete for Health and Performance. Gatorade Sports Science Institute, October 19, 2002, Philadelphia, Pa.
22. Engles, H. J., et al. (2001). Effects of ginseng supplementation on supramaximal exercise performance and short-term recovery. Journal of Strength and Conditioning Research, 15, 3, 290-295.
23. Engels, H. J. et al. (1997). No ergogenic effects of ginseng (Panax ginseng) during graded maximal aerobic exercise. Journal of the American Dietetic Association, 97, 10, 1110-1115.
24. Gibala, M. J. et al. (2000). Amino acids, proteins and exercise performance. Sports science exchange roundtable 42, volume 11, # 2. Gatorade Sports Science Institute. http://www.gssiweb.com
25. Grant K. E., Chandler R. M., Castle A. L., Ivy J. L. (1997). Chromium and exercise training: effect

on obese women. Medicine and Science in Sports and Exercise, 29, 8, 992-998.

26. Groff, J. L., Gropper, S. S., Hunt, S. M. (1995). Advanced Nutrition and Human Metabolism, 2nd edt. West Publishing Company.

27. Heyward, V. (1991). Advanced Fitness Assessment & Exercise Prescription 2nd edt. Human Kinetics.

28. Howley, E. T. & Franks, B. D. (1997). Health Fitness InstructorsHandbook, 3rd edt. Human Kinetics.

29. Jellin, J. M. Betz, F., Hitchens, K. (1999). Natural Medicines Comprehensive Database. Therapeutic Research Faculty.

30. Kleiner, S. (1998). Power Eating. Human Kinetics.

31. Kreider. R. B. (1999). Dietary supplements and the promotion of muscle growth with resistance exercise. Sports Medicine, 27, 2, 97-110.

32. Kundrat, S. (2002). Nutritional nuances for athletes in stop-and-go sports. Presented at: Inside the Athlete: Fueling the Athlete for Health and Performance. Gatorade Sports Science Institute, October 19, 2002, Philadelphia, Pa.

33. Lockner D.W. et al. (2000). Comparison of air-displacement plethysmography, hydrodensitometry, and dual X-ray absorptiometry for assessing body composition of children 10 to 18 years of age. Annals of the New York Academy of Science, 904, 72-78.

34. Maddalozzo, G. F..et al. (2002). Concurrent validity of the BOD POD and dual energy x-ray absorptiometry techniques for assessing body composition in young women. Journal of the American Dietetic Association, 102,11,1677-1679.

35. Maughan, R. J. Leiper, J. P. (1993). Post exercise dehydration in man. Effects of voluntary intake of four different beverages,. Medicine and Science in Sports and Exercise, 25 (suppl), S2-S10.

36. McArdle, W. D., Katch, F. I., Katch, V. L. (1999). Sport & Exercise Nutrition. Lippincott, Williams & Wilkins.

37. Murray, R. et al. (1999). International Journal of Sports Nutrition, 9, 263-274.

38. Neiman, D. C. (1998). The Exercise Health Connection. Human Kinetics.

39. Nissen, S. K. Abumrad, N. N. (1997). Nutritional role of the leucine metabolite B-hydroxy B-methylbutyrate (HMB). Journal of Nutritional Biochemistry, 8, 300-311.

40. Pieralisi, G., Ripari, P., Vecchiet, L. (1991). Effects of a standardized ginseng extract combined with dimethylaminoethanol bitartrate, vitamins, minerals, and trace elements on physical performance during exercise. Clinical Therapeutics, 13, 3, 373-82.

41. Powers, S. K., Howley, E. T. (1990). Exercise Physiology, 2nd edition Brown & Benchmark.

42. Rankin, J. W. (1997). Glycemic index and exercise metabolism. Sports science exchange #64, volume 10 #1. Gatorade Sports Science Institute http://www.gssiweb.com

43. Rasmussen, B. B. (2000). Androstenedione does not stimulate muscle protein anabolism in young healthy men. Journal of Clinical Endocrinology and Metabolism, 85,1, 55-59.

44. Reimers, K. J. (2001). Glycemic index. Can you use it? Strength and Conditioning Journal, 23, 5,69-70.

45. Reimers, K. J. (1999). High-protein diets, right for athletes? Strength and Conditioning Journal, 21, 4. 34-35.

46. Rimm, E.B., et al. (1996). Vegetable, fruit, and cereal fiber intake and risk of coronary heart disease among men. Journal of the American Medical Association, 275, 6, 447-451.

47. Salmeron, J. (1997). Dietary fiber, glycemic load, and risk of non-insulin- dependent diabetes mellitus in women. Journal of the American Medical Association, 277, 6, 472-477.

48. Salonen, J. T. et al. (1992). High stored iron levels are associated with excess risk of myocardial infarction in eastern Finnish men. Circulation, 86, 803-811.

49. Shekelle, P. et al. (2003). The Rand Report. Ephedra and Ephedrine for Weight Loss and Athletic Performance Enhancement: Clinical Efficacy and Side Effects. Evidence Report/Technology Assessment Number 76. AHRQ Publication No. 03-E022.

50. Solomon, P. R., Adams, F., Silver, A., Zimmer, J., DeVeaux, R. (2002). Ginkgo for memory enhancement: a randomized controlled trial. JAMA, 21, 288, 7, 835-40.

51. Tedd, L et al. (1998). Controlling Blood Lipids. Part 1: A practical role for diet and exercise. Physician and Sports Medicine, 26, 10.

52. Tyler, V. (1993). The Honest Herbal. Pharmaceutical Produces Press.

53. Utter, A.C. et al. (2003). Evaluation of air displacement for assessing body composition of collegiate wrestlers. Medicine and Science in Sports and Exercise, 35,3, 500-505.

54. van Dongen M. C., (2000). The efficacy of ginkgo for elderly people with dementia and age-associated memory impairment: new results of a randomized clinical trial. American Geriatric Society, 48, 10, 1183-1194.

55. Vescovi, J. D. et al. (2002). Evaluation of the BOD POD for estimating percent fat in female college athletes. Journal of Strength and Conditioning Research, 16, 4, 599-605.

56. Vescovi, J.D. et al. (2001). Evaluation of the BOD POD for estimating percentage body fat in a heterogeneous group of adult humans. European Journal of Applied Physiology, 85, 3-4, 326-332.

57. Villani, R.G. et al. (2000). L-Carnitine supplementation combined with aerobic training does not promote weight loss in moderately obese women. International Journal of Sports Nutrition and Exercise Metabolism, 10, 2,199-207.

58. Volek, J. S. (1997). Testosterone and cortisol in relationship to dietary nutrients and resistance training. Journal of Applied Physiology, 82, 1, 49-54.

59. Wang, X. D. & Russell, R. M. (1999). Procarcinogenic and anticarcinogenic effects of beta-carotene. Nutritional Reviews. 57, 263-272.

60. Williams, M. (1998). The Ergogenics Edge. Human Kinetics.

61. Williams, M. et al. (1999). Creatine: The Power Supplement. Human Kinetics.

62. Inserra, P. et al. (1999). Immune function in elderly smokers and non-smokers improves during supplementation with fruit and vegetable extracts. Integrative Medicine, 2,1, 3-10.

63. Smith, M. (1999). Supplements with fruit and vegetable extracts may decrease DNA damage in the peripheral lymphocytes of an elderly population. Nutrition Research, 19, 10,1507-1518.

64. Van Duyn et al. (2000). Overview of health benefits of fruit and vegetable consumption for the dietetic professional: selected literature. Journal of the American Dietetic Association, 100, 1511-1521.

65. Wise, J. (1996). Changes in plasma carotenoids, alpha tocopherol and lipid peroxide levels in response to supplementation with concentrated fruit and vegetable extracts: a pilot study. Current Therapeutic Research, 57, 6, 445-461.

66. Shabert JK et al. (1999). Glutamine-antioxidant supplementation increases body cell mass in AIDS patients with weight loss: a randomized, double-blind controlled trial. Nutrition 15,860-864.

67. Tepaske R et al. (2001). Effect of preoperative oral immune-enhancing nutritional supplement on patients at high risk of infection after cardiac surgery: a randomized placebo-controlled trial. Lancet 358,696-701.

68. Hanis T et al. (1989). Effects of dietary trans-fatty acids on reproductive performance of Wistar rats. British Journal of Nutrition, 61,3,519-529.

69. Journal of the American Dietetic Association (2000). Position statement. Nutrition and athletic performance: Position of the American Dietetic Association, Dietitians of Canada, and the American College of Sports Medicine. Journal of the American Dietetic Association, 100, 1543-1556.

70. No authors listed. Glycemic Index: What is It? American Dietetic Association March 19 2004. www.eatright.org/cps/rde/xchg/ada/hs.xsl/home_4456_ENU_HTML.htm (accessed 10/2/05).

71. Hidgon J (2003). Glycemic Index and Glycemic load. Linus Pauling Institute. http://lpi.oregonstate.edu/infocenter/foods/grains/gigl.html (accessed 10/2/05).

72. Martin WF et al. (2005). Dietary protein intake and renal function. Nutrition and Metabolism, Available at Biomed Central http://www.nutritionandmetabolism.com/content/2/1/25 (accessed 10/4/05)

73. Belury M (2002). Beyond the Headlines: Not all trans fatty acids are alike: what consumers may lose when they oversimplify nutrition facts. Journal of the American Dietetic Association, 102,11,1606-1607

74. Shabert JK (1999). Glutamine-antioxidant supplementation increases body cell mass in AIDS patients with weight loss: a randomized, double-blind controlled trial. Nutrition, 15,860-864.

75. Antonio J et al. (2002). The effects of high-dose glutamine ingestion on weightlifting performance. Journal of Strength Condoning Research, 16,157–160.

76. Clark RH et al. (2000). Nutritional treatment for acquired immunodeficiency virus-associated wasting using beta-hydroxy beta-methylbutyrate, glutamine, and arginine: a randomized, double-blind, placebo-controlled study. Journal of Parenteral and Enteral Nutrition, 24,3,133-1339.

77. Miller ER et al. (2005). Meta-analysis: High-dosage vitamin E supplementation may increase all-cause mortality. Annals of Internal Medicine, 142, 60520-60553.

78. No authors listed (Feb 2001). How much protein is enough. Consumer Reports on Health. Consumerreports.org

79. McNaughton LR et al. (1999). Sodium bicarbonate can be used as an ergogenic aid in high-intensity, competitive cycle ergometry of 1 h duration. European Journal of Applied Physiology and Occupational Physiology, 80,1,64-69.

80. Virtamo J et al. (2003). Incidence of cancer and mortality following alpha-tocopherol and beta-carotene supplementation: a postintervention follow-up. JAMA,290,476-485.

81. Davidson G et al. (2005). Influence of acute vitamin C and/or carbohydrate ingestion on hormonal, cytokine and immune responses to prolonged exercise. International Journal of Sport Nutrition and Exercise Metabolism, 15,465-479.

82. Benvenga S et al. (2000). Carnitine is a naturally occurring inhibitor of thyroid hormone nuclear uptake. Thyroid, 10, 1043–1050.

83. Wald DS et al. (2001). Randomized trial of folic acid supplementation and serum homocysteine levels. Archives of Internal Medicine, 161,695-700.

84. Bischoff-Ferrari HA et al. (2004). Effect of Vitamin D on falls: a meta-analysis. JAMA, 291,1999-2006.

85. Boehnke Cet al. (2004). High-dose riboflavin treatment is efficacious in migraine prophylaxis: an open study in a tertiary care centre. European Journal of Neurology, 11,475-477.

86. Garg R (1999). Niacin treatment increases plasma homocyst(e)ine levels. American Heart Journal 138,1082-1087.

87. Cumming RG et al. (2000).Diet and cataract: the Blue Mountains Eye Study. Ophthalmology, 10,450-456.

88. Visalli N et al. (1999). A multi-centre randomized trial of two different doses of nicotinamide in patients with recent-onset type 1 diabetes (the IMDIAB VI). Diabetes/Metabolism Research and Reviews, 15,181-185.

89. Zhao XQ et al. (1993). Effects of intensive lipid-lowering therapy on the coronary arteries of asymptomatic subjects with elevated apolipoprotein B. Circulation, 88,2744-2753.

90. Brown BG (2001). Simvastatin and niacin, antioxidant vitamins, or the combination for the prevention of coronary disease. New England Journal of Medicine, 345,1583-1593..

91. Friso S et al. (2001). Low circulating vitamin B(6) is associated with elevation of the inflammation marker C-reactive protein independently of plasma homocysteine levels. Circulation, 103,2788-2791.

92. Eros E et al. (1998). Epileptogenic activity of folic acid after drug induces SLE (folic acid and epilepsy). European Journal of Obstetrics, Gynecology, and Reproductive Biology, 80,75-77.

93. Sheldon, M (2002). UC Berkeley Wellness Foods A to Z. Rebus.

94. Higdon J (2004). Vitamin C. Linus Pauling Institute. www.lip.origonstate.edu (accessed 4/ 19/05).

95. McAlindon TE et al. (1996). Do antioxidant micronutrients protect against the development and progression of knee osteoarthritis? Arthritis and Rheumatology, 39,648-656.

96. Simon JA et al. (2001). Relation of ascorbic acid to bone mineral density and self-reported fractures among US adults. American Journal of Epidemiology, 154,427-433.

97. Peters EM et al. (2001). Vitamin C supplementation attenuates the increases in circulating cortisol, adrenaline and anti-inflammatory polypeptides following ultramarathon running. International Journal of Sport Nutrition and Exercise Metabolism, 22,537-543.

98. Labriola D et al. (1999). Possible interactions between dietary antioxidants and chemotherapy. Oncology, 13:1003-1008.

99. Iso H et al. (1999). Prospective study of calcium, potassium, and magnesium intake and risk of stroke in women. Stroke, 30,1772-1779.

100. Zemel MB et al. (2004). Calcium and dairy acceleration of weight and fat loss during energy restriction in obese adults. Obesity Research, 12,582-580.

101. Guerrero-Romero F et al. (2004). Oral magnesium supplementation improves insulin sensitivity in non-diabetic subjects with insulin resistance. A double-blind placebo-controlled randomized trial. Diabetes and Metabolism, 30,253-258.

102. Jee SH, Miller ER 3rd, Guallar E, et al. (2002).The effect of magnesium supplementation on blood pressure: a meta-analysis of randomized clinical trials. American Journal of Hypertension, 15,691-696.

103. Guerrero-Romero F (2002). Relationship between serum magnesium levels and C-reactive protein concentration, in non-diabetic, non-hypertensive obese subjects. International Journal of Obesity and Related Metabolic Disorders, 26,469-474.

104. Dobson AW (2004). Manganese neurotoxicity. Annals of the New York Academy of Sciences, 1012,115-128.

105. Hidgon J (2003). Phosphorus. Linus Pauling Institute. http://lpi.oregonstate.edu/infocenter/minerals/phosphorus/index.html (accessed 10/28/05)

106. Hidgon J (2003). Potassium. Linus Pauling Institute. http://lpi.oregonstate.edu/infocenter/minerals/potassium/index.html (accessed 10/28/05).

107. Food and Nutrition Board, Institute of Medicine. Dietary Reference Intakes for Vitamin C, Vitamin E, Selenium, and Carotenoids. Washington, DC: National Academy Press, 2000. Available at: http://www.nap.edu/books/0309069351/html/

108. Prasad AS et al. (1996). Zinc status and serum testosterone levels of healthy adults. Nutrition, 12,5,344-348.

109. Higdon J (2003). Zinc. Linus Pauling Institute. http://lpi.oregonstate.edu/infocenter/minerals/zinc/index.html (accessed 7/7/05).

110. Ibs HK et al. (2003). Zinc-altered immune function. Journal of Nutrition, 133,1452S-1456S.

111. van Loon LJ et al. (2003). Amino acid ingestion strongly enhances insulin secretion in patients with long-term type 2 diabetes. Diabetes Care, 26,625-630.

112. Stearns, DM et al. (1995), Chromium(III) picolinate produces chromosome damage inChinese hamster ovary cells. FASEB Journal, 9,15,1643-8.

113. Kroboth PD et al. (1999). DHEA and DHEA-S: A review. Journal of Clinical Pharmacology, 39,327-348.

114 Villareal DT et al. (2004). Effect of DHEA on abdominal fat and insulin action in elderly women and men. Journal of the American Medical Association, 292,2243-2248.

115. Benjamin J et al. (2001). A case of cerebral haemorrhage-can Ginkgo biloba be implicated? Journal of Postgraduate Medicine, 77,904,112-113.

116. Richy F et al. (2003). Structural and symptomatic efficacy of glucosamine and chondroitin in knee osteoarthritis: a comprehensive meta-analysis. Archives of Internal Medicine, 163,1514-1522.

117. Panton LB et al. (2000).Nutritional supplementation of the leucine metabolite beta-hydroxy-beta-methylbutyrate (hmb) during resistance training. Nutrition, 16,734-739.

118. Metabolic Technologies homepage http://www.mettechinc.com/ (accessed 3/17/04).

119. Bo-Linn GW et al. (1983). Starch blockers--their effect on calorie absorption from a high-starch meal. New England Journal of Medicine, 307, 23, 1413-1416.

120. Hollenbeck CB et al. (1983). Effects of a commercial starch blocker preparation on carbohydrate digestion and absorption: in vivo and in vitro studies. American Journal of Clinical Nutrition, 38,4, 498-503.

121. Umoren J. et al. (1992). Commercial soybean starch blocker consumption: impact on weight gain and on copper, lead and zinc status of rats. Plant Foods for Human Nutrition, 42, 2, 135-142.

122. Schnirring L (2000). When to suspect muscle dysmorphia. The Physician and Sports Medicine, 28,12, http://www.physsportsmed.com/issues/2000/12_00/news.htm (accessed 11/4/05).

123. Broeder CE (1997). Assessing body composition before and after resistance or endurance training. Medicine and Science in Sports and Exercise, 29,5, 705-712.

124. Foster DG et al. (2003). A randomized trial for a low-carbohydrate diet for obesity. New England Journal of Medicine, 348,21,2082-2090.

125. Dansinger DL et al. (2005). Comparison of the Atkins, Ornish, Weight Watchers and Zone diets for weight loss and heart disease risk reduction, Journal of the American Medical Association, 293,43-53.

126. Guyton AC et al. (1996). Textbook of Medical Physiology, 9th edition.

127. Rating the diet books. Center for Science in the Public Interest. May 2000

128. Brown TB (2004). Exertional Rhabdomyolysis. Physician and Sports Medicine 34,4 physsportsmed.com

129. Hultman E et al. (1996). Muscle creatine loading in men. Journal of Applied Physiology, 81,1,232-237.

130. Rawson ES (2004). Effects of repeated creatine supplementation on muscle, plasma, and urine creatine levels. Journal of Strength and Conditioning Research 18,1,162-167.

131. National Heart, Lung, and Blood Institute, National Institutes of Health (2000). The Practical Guide: Identification, Evaluation, and Treatment of Overweight and Obesity in Adults (NIH Publication No. 00-4084). www.nhlbi.nih.gov/guidelines/obesity/prctgd_c.pdf

132. Shai, I et al. (2008). Weight loss with a low-carbohydrate, Mediterranean or low fat diet. New England Journal of Medicine, 17,359,229-241.

133. ACSM's Guidelines for Exercise Testing and Prescription, 7th edt. (2006). Lippincott, Williams & Wilkins.

134. Phillips, SM (2007). A critical examination of dietary protein requirements, benefits and excess in athletes. International Journal of Sports Nutrition and Exercise Metabolism, 17,S58-S76.

135. Bjelakovic G et al. (2007). Mortality in randomized trials of antioxidant supplements for primary and secondary prevention: systematic review and meta-analysis. Journal of the American Medical Association, 297, 842-857.

136. Feskanich D et al. (2002). Vitamin A intake and hip fractures among postmenopausal women. Journal of the American Medical Association, 287,47-54.

137. Sano M et al. (1997). A controlled trial of selegiline, alpha-tocopherol, or both as treatment for Alzheimer's disease. The Alzheimer's Disease Cooperative Study. New England Journal of Medicine, 336,1216-1222.

138. Masaki KH et al. (2000). Association of vitamin E and C supplement use with cognitive function and dementia in elderly men. Neurology, 54,1265-1272.

139. Lappe JM et al. (2007). Vitamin D and calcium supplementation reduces cancer risk: results of a randomized trial. American Journal of Clinical Nutrition, 85,1586-1591.

140. Wortsman J et al. (2000). Decreased bioavailability of vitamin D in obesity. American Journal of Clinical Nutrition, 72,690-693.

141. Esmarck B et al. (2001). Timing of postexercise protein intake is important for muscle hypertrophy with resistance training in elderly humans. Journal of Applied Physiology 535,1,301-311.

142. Athletes and Protein Intake. Today's Dietitian. Vol 16 No. 6 P.22. June 2014

143. The Alkaline Diet: Is There Evidence That an Alkaline pH Diet Benefits Health? J Environ Public Health. 2012; 2012: 727630.

144. ABO Genotype, 'Blood-Type' Diet and Cardiometabolic Risk Factors PLoS ONE, 2014; 9 (1): e84749.

Index

About Joe Cannon

Joe Cannon, is an exercise physiologist, personal trainer, and health educator. He holds an MS degree in Exercise Science and a BS degree in Chemistry & Biology. A dynamic and motivational speaker who specializes presenting scientific information in easy to understand terms, Joe has been a member of the AAAI/ISMA education facility since 1995, lecturing on the topics of sports nutrition, supplements health, and personal fitness training.

He has two websites:

1. Joe-Cannon.com is where he writes about personal training, health, and wellness.

2. Supplement-Geek.com is where he writes user-friendly, science-based reviews of dietary supplements.

Joe can be reached directly at either of his websites.

Books by Joe Cannon

1. *Personal Fitness Training: Beyond The Basics*: Outshine your competition! Joe Cannon reviews not only the science of exercise, but also how to apply that knowledge to the real world. This book also covers real life issues that fitness professionals encounter each day. Essentially, a textbook that cuts out the technical stuff most trainers don't need while focusing on what they should know, the emphasis is to not only help you be certified, but also be a **qualified** personal trainer as well. This is the companion book to *Nutrition Essentials*.

2. *Personal Trainer Practice Test*: This test was created to show trainers the knowledge necessary to pass a certification test and be a good personal trainer. This ebook can be downloaded immediately from Joe Cannon's website.

3. **Rhabdo: The Scary Side Effect Of Exercise You've Never heard Of**. Learn what can happen when you exercise too much. This book may save your life!

4. *Nutritional Supplements*: A no-nonsense scientific review of 119 vitamins, minerals, herbs, and other supplements. This book cuts through the hype and deciphers what works and what doesn't as well as providing unbiased information about supplement side effects that most people have never heard before. An eye-opening must-read for everyone who takes supplements. Easy to read with over 900 references, this book is the culmination of over 15 years of Joe Cannon's study and investigation of dietary supplements.

5. *Nutrition Essentials*: An information-packed nutrition and sports nutrition guidebook that was designed specifically to address the needs of fitness professionals as well as to help them study and prepare for *any* sports nutrition certification. *Nutrition Essentials* is the companion text to Joe's book on Personal Fitness Training.

6. *Personal Trainer's Big Book of Questions and Answers*: This book provides quick and accurate answers to over 135 exercise, nutrition, and general health questions that fitness professionals are asked every day. No need to search for the answers to people's questions anymore. They are right here! This is an e-book that can be downloaded immediately from Joe Cannon's website.

For more information or to order any of these books, visit www.Joe-Cannon.com.

25033455R00085

Made in the USA
San Bernardino, CA
15 October 2015